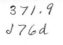

Dyslexia in the Classroom

Second Edition

Dale R. Jordan

Jordan-Adams Learning Center
Oklahoma City, Oklahoma

Charles E. Merrill Publishing Company
A Bell & Howell Company
Columbus, Ohio 43216

19,800

This book was set in Times Roman and Bodoni italic.
The production editor was Jan Hall.
The cover was prepared by Will Chenoweth.

Published by
Charles E. Merrill Publishing Company
A Bell & Howell Company
Columbus, Ohio 43216

International Standard Book Number: 0–675–08466–0

Library of Congress Catalog Card Number: 76-49375

1 2 3 4 5 6 7 8 9 10—81 80 79 78 77

Printed in the United States of America

Preface

The original conception for *Dyslexia in the Classroom* grew out of my contacts with prison inmates, juvenile delinquents, and school dropouts—those heartbreaking casualties who don't make it in our standard social and educational systems. When the first edition of this book appeared, almost no published information was available concerning the relationships between delinquency and learning disability. Suddenly in the mid-1970's a great deal of attention became focused on this costly social problem. As the second edition of *Dyslexia in the Classroom* reaches the public, more than 40 research projects have reported learning disability syndromes in 71 to 85 percent of all convicted male felons in our penal systems.[1]

In spite of mounting evidence that learning disability is active among us, many educational leaders still deny its prevalence or even its existence. Dyslexia is often derided as a myth, or worse, as a fad promoted by private clinics at inflated fees. Classroom teachers, harassed social workers, and peace officers who deal with illiterate adolescents know that *something* is not alright with these young people. Those of us working closely with delinquents and felons see the pathetic consequences of unrecognized and untreated learning problems.

More and more professionals in all fields are speaking of *dyslexia*, when the term applies. No doubt a better term will someday appear, but until it does, an effort must be made to remediate the symbol confusion found in every classroom in the nation. Academic debate serves as a vital role in achieving clarity, but teachers and diagnosticians cannot wait for consensus at the top. Steps must be taken now to help the patient even before the doctors agree upon cause and nomenclature.

This book is not an attempt to set the experts straight regarding learning disability. Instead, this book is intended for grass-roots professionals who have neither time nor opportunity for specialized study of learning disabilities. My purpose is to give simple, trustworthy guidelines for identifying specific kinds of learning problems and then to offer workable suggestions for solving many of these problems in the classroom. To bring this sort of fire down from Olympus, I must give it all a name. That name, as defined in the following chapters, is *dyslexia*.

Dale R. Jordan, Ph.D.
Oklahoma City, Oklahoma
Spring, 1977

---

[1] "The Link Between Learning Disabilities and Juvenile Delinquency: Current Theory and Knowledge," available from the American Institute for Research, 3301 New Mexico Avenue, N. W., Washington, D. C. 20016.

Contents

chapter 4   **Dysgraphia in the Classroom**   **50**

chapter 5   **Correcting Visual Dyslexia in the Classroom**   **69**

chapter 6   **Correcting Auditory Dyslexia in the Classroom**   **90**

chapter 7 Correcting Dysgraphia in the Classroom 116

chapter 8   Distinguishing Dyslexia from
                    Other Disabilities   133

chapter 1

Three Faces of Dyslexia

TEACHERS HAVE OBSERVED A MYSTERIOUS DILEMMA IN THE CLASSROOM for many years. Certain intelligent children never learn to read, write, spell, or compute at grade level, no matter what methods of instruction are used. Diligent teachers have always sensed that this puzzling failure is not due to pupil laziness alone. In fact, many of these failing pupils are the most industrious members of the class. Nor can their failure be attributed to stupidity or defective intellect. These particular nonreaders usually exhibit brightness in oral-language fluency. What, then, is the matter? Because they lack satisfactory explanations or solutions, most teachers have assigned these children to the next higher grade, hoping they will someday outgrow their learning limitations.

For many years educators have known that millions of school children fail to reach the proficiency of their grade level in reading, writing, spelling, and arithmetic. The percentages of failure fluctuate according to the degree of teacher enthusiasm, freshness of methodology, and various other factors in the teaching-learning process. A unique, hard-core failure group persists, however, within the student population. Regardless of the materials or methods used or the amount of teacher stimulus, these unique children remain frustrated when attempting to master symbols and standard nomenclature. These children are identified as dyslexic. It appears that ten to fifteen percent of the school age population experiences this strange inability to handle language symbols, in spite of good mental ability, comfortable economic status, or instructional efforts within the classroom (42).

What is Dyslexia?

Many professionals have attempted to define this educational deficiency. Great differences exist between various definitions and philosophies.

1

Many years ago Dr. Samuel Orton, a neurologist, coined the term *strephosymbolia,* which he defined as "twisted symbols" (31). He attempted to classify the behavior of children who perceive letters and words backwards, upside down, or in a distorted fashion. Later another term appeared, *alexia,* which designates the mysterious inability of intelligent persons to recognize printed words. Alexia, or "word blindness," is still widely used by professionals in many fields.

During the past three decades other labels for the chronic nonreader have evolved: *dyslexia, specific dyslexia, minimal brain dysfunction,* or *minimal cerebral damage.* Special designations for related learning disorders have appeared: *agraphia* and *dysgraphia,* for disorders in handwriting; *agnosia* and *dysgnosia,* for disorders in remembering specific language factors; and *acalculia* and *dyscalculia,* for faulty arithmetic perception. Each of these terms has a useful meaning (see Glossary). But the high incidence of overlapping between professional disciplines has resulted in ambiguity. There is presently no single set of terms which is satisfactory for general communication among those who treat language disorders (1).

A useful diagnostic term that is gaining acceptability is dyslexia. Two major professional camps claim priority for this label, however. On the one hand, medical disciplines infer a physical disability as the cause of reading failure. As used by most physicians, dyslexia denotes a set of behaviors caused by brain damage, or at the least by brain dysfunction (4, 7, 9, 17, 31, 49). Brain damage or dysfunction means that brain tissue has been destroyed by physical injury, or that certain brain systems only partially function because of accident, disease, or faulty body chemistry. Diagnosis is usually made by means of an EEG, or brain wave evaluation. Medication is frequently prescribed to tone down nervousness or hyperactivity in the dyslexic child. Certain clinics prescribe rigorous physical training, called patterning, in an effort to stimulate damaged or malfunctioning brain centers into organized activity.

On the other hand, many researchers believe that dyslexia is not a matter of brain injury, but is the result of dormant or undeveloped learning centers in the brain structure. The problem is defined in terms of the child's classroom behavior. According to this definition, dyslexia can be corrected by overteaching specific skills, such as letter formation, phonics, handwriting, and spelling (10, 21, 27, 28, 32, 36).

Although those who hold this point of view often welcome medication for hyperactive children, they basically believe that dyslexia is correctable through the stimulation of inactive brain centers. This process is sometimes described as imprinting, or training the child's perceptual processes through exaggerated drills.

Many other educators who have no strong opinions either way so far as cause is concerned are caught between these opposite poles of view. Their primary concern is simply to identify the deficient behavior, outline appropriate instructional procedures, and teach dyslexics to function in language situations. Since the causes of dyslexia are not definitely known, if educators waited for them to be definitely determined before acting, they would see millions of semiliterates passing unprepared into adult life in the meantime.

Regardless of its causes, dyslexia is a very real factor in everyday classroom situations. Whether Johnny's brain was damaged at birth actually has little bearing upon his success or failure in Mrs. Jones's Grade Two reading circle on Monday. And whether or not Mary's inability to distinguish "bed" from "bid" was caused by an oxygen loss when she nearly drowned three years ago has no classroom significance as she struggles to cope with next Friday's spelling test. The immediate concern for teachers is what can be done now, within the context of school limitations, to help Johnny and Mary become independent, literate individuals.

Kinds of Dyslexia

As used in this book, the term dyslexia is defined as *the inability to process language symbols.* This means that the child cannot cope with school tasks involving the discrete (separate) sounds of spoken language, or the written symbols of the language. As is true in all cases of disability, no two children exhibit the same sets of symptoms. In the same way, no two children will be handicapped to the same degree. Dyslexia is seen as a continuum, ranging from rather mild forms of symbol confusion to complex syndromes of disabilities.

In traditional classroom methodologies it has been assumed that all children can master three kinds of language symbols: oral-aural symbols used in speaking and listening; printed symbols used in reading; and written symbols used in handwriting. Educators have also assumed that all children are capable of automatically progressing from left to right across the page, as well as from top to bottom down the page. Publishers have produced educational materials fashioned upon these assumptions. Through the years virtually no one has questioned whether these assumptions are in fact valid. Recent concern over the millions of nonreaders in our schools has caused a reappraisal of these expectations of learning (14, 15, 19, 21, 27, 28, 32, 36, 43).

For perhaps fifteen percent of our population, these basic assumptions about learning to read are not true. Dyslexic children do not master language symbols, and they do not perceive left to right and top to bottom. Some dyslexics cannot handle the processes involved in translating spoken language into written symbol forms, often referred to as "encoding." This means that such children cannot put what they hear into an accurate written code. Other dyslexics have difficulty translating symbols into meaning. Thus they are unable to "decode" what they see in printed form. Still others cannot express themselves in writing because they cannot remember how to make specific letter forms correctly. These students are unable to control directionality of written symbols, which results in unacceptable handwriting. These forms of disability are complicated by the tendency to perceive symbols backwards, upside down, and in scrambled sequence. Traditional assumptions do not apply to a sizable minority of the student population.

The major difficulty in the classroom, however, is that few children are handicapped by only one form of dyslexia. Two or more kinds of this perceptual loss usually exist in dyslexic children. These complexes of perceptual handicaps make it all the more difficult for the disability to be corrected. In fact, severe cases of dyslexia require special clinical treatment which a regular classroom cannot possibly provide. It is essential that teachers be able to screen their pupils in order to make the necessary referrals for those children that need specialized help. Contrary to general belief, however, most of the dyslexic population can be treated within the usual classroom structure, if teachers can make certain adjustments in assignments and learning procedures.

Visual Dyslexia

The most prevalent form of dyslexic handicap is that of visual dyslexia. This is basically the inability to translate printed language symbols into meaning (see Glossary). Visual dyslexia has little to do with vision itself (see Chapter 8). Children with severe visual impairment are not dyslexic because of loss of sight. Visual dyslexia is not a matter of seeing poorly; it is a matter of not interpreting accurately what is seen.

Most visual dyslexics see certain letters backwards and upside down. To read whole words in the context of a sentence is a jumbled process for such a child. Not only does he perceive individual letters incorrectly, but he also sees parts of words in reverse. When these faults are at work during reading tasks, the child has a disorganized, meaningless, and frustrating experience. Consequently, he does everything in his power to avoid reading.

For example, Mike, who is handicapped by visual dyslexia, is asked to read the following paragraph silently:

> Down the cold, dark stairs crept the man in the black coat. Closer he came, closer and closer. Asleep in their blankets, Dan and Pete were unaware of their danger.

Because of reversals, transpositions, and failure to perceive minimal cues (see Glossary), this is Mike's perception of the paragraph the first time he reads it:

> Now the could, back stars keep the man in the dalk coat. Colser he come, colser and colser sheeping the dantes anD and deer wore nuraw for the bang.

The teacher, who is unaware of the nature of Mike's reading disability, has made an issue of subvocalizing. She snaps her fingers and says "Shhhhhh!" when Mike mutters as he reads. The teacher does not realize that, by cutting off the oral-aural (speaking-listening) channels, she has made it impossible for the boy to check his visual impressions against what is meaningful to him through hearing. The result is complete nonsense for Mike, and he flunks still another comprehension quiz because of his silent reading. Had he been allowed to mumble the words, thus checking them against his listening vocabulary, he could have slowly worked out the meaning of the passage.

Because of this sort of scrambled perception, visual dyslexics are forced to work very slowly. This slowness is a factor usually misunderstood by teachers. If the typical pupil in Mike's class can digest the above passage in three minutes, it will take him at least fifteen minutes, as a rule. The demands for speed in reading and writing are being increased by the pressures of the modern curriculum, but visual dyslexics are incapable of such speed. When they are placed with impatient instructors who do not understand their problems, children like Mike have no way of coping with their assigned reading tasks.

Because the visual dyslexic has such a constant problem handling information in sequence, he usually experiences difficulty with basic arithmetic. Learning to add, subtract, multiply, and divide involves frequent changes in direction that contradict the left-to-right, top-to-bottom orientation stressed in reading and writing. To add, Mike must start at the right side of the problem and work downward, then carry right-to-left to the next column. In simple first grade work this orientation is not difficult. When more complex addition problems are introduced, he becomes confused by this new directionality which is opposite to (backwards from) the emphasis placed in reading and writing. To subtract or multiply, Mike must start at the bottom right, exactly opposite from the orientation for other paper/pencil work during the school day. In subtracting and multiplying he must work bottom-to-top, right-to-left. Long division involves a complex pattern of beginning left-to-right, then top-to-bottom, then bottom-to-top and right-to-left, then back to left-to-right again. If reading this description makes your adult-head swirl, you can imagine the confusion Mike faces when he is under pressure to hurry through arithmetic computation. He constantly loses direction and is forced to start over. When he is not given enough time to correct his directionality, he becomes enormously frustrated and confused.

Visual dyslexics are generally handicapped in any situation which requires them to comprehend sequence. Pupils like Mike cannot remember the order of the months of the year, days of the week, multiplication tables, or even the day, month, and year of their birth. Mike's parents and teachers have fussed about his habit of "forgetting" to do routine chores, or to carry out a set of instructions. The problem is not one of laziness or rebellion on his part, as a rule. He simply does not perceive serial relationships. His comprehension of household duties, as well as classroom tasks, is as scrambled as his perception of printed symbols. It is unfortunate that such children are regarded as irresponsible. The fact is they are confused.

Of the three forms of dyslexia commonly found in classrooms, visual dyslexia is the most easily corrected. Fortunately Mike can identify discrete (separate) sounds of speech, making it relatively easy for him to learn phonics. His major handicap is the inability to visualize printed symbols in correct sequence or position. Through appropriate drills he can learn to perceive printed symbols accurately, although he will probably remain a slow reader all of his life. Gradually he can learn to identify sequence in his environment, thus reducing his conflict with adult expectations. His greatest enemies are pressure for speed and pressure for quantity of work produced. If he is given proper allowances for his limitations, Mike can become a strong student; he can even achieve advanced scholastic standing. Many adults have gained remarkable success in spite of dyslexia.

Auditory Dyslexia

The most difficult form of dyslexia to correct is the inability to perceive the discrete (separate) sounds of spoken language. Auditory dyslexia has little to do with hearing acuity. Most auditory dyslexics have normal hearing, so far as can be determined by audiometer tests. The basic handicap is similar to that of "tone deafness" toward music, a condition which spoils music appreciation for many adults. Because the dyslexic cannot identify small differences between vowel sounds or consonant sounds, he is unable to associate specific sounds with their printed symbols. Consequently he is very poor at spelling and composition. Traditional phonics instruction is almost meaningless to most auditory dyslexics. They simply cannot identify the discrete variations of speech sounds, nor do the rules and generalizations make sense.

For example, Mary is handicapped in this way. The seriousness of her problem is illustrated most clearly when she must write without receiving help from others. Without being aware of Mary's perceptual limitations, her teacher has chosen to give a dictation test. While speaking clearly and slowly, the teacher dictates: "What kind of celebration did the Pilgrims have to show their thankfulness to God?" Mary's task is to encode this sentence with no help from anyone else.

As usual her teacher becomes annoyed when Mary asks for the fifth time that the sentence be repeated. This need for repetition is characteristic of auditory dyslexics who are never sure that they have heard correctly. As she struggles to write the sentence, Mary is acutely aware of her teacher's disapproving frown. Under these conditions, this is the best the child can do: "What cid of selbarshun dind the Plegms hev too sow tere takfulnis too Gode?"

At her very best working speed, Mary requires from three to five minutes to encode a simple dictated sentence. Before she can finish one item, her teacher moves on to the next. As usual Mary completes only two or three of the ten dictated sentences. Thus she has met failure again, something she has come to expect.

Children like Mary are at a serious disadvantage in standardized testing. The three most widely used intelligence tests for placing children in special classes are the Peabody Picture Vocabulary Test, the Wechsler Intelligence Scale for Children (WISC), and the Stanford-Binet Intelligence Scale. These tests involve careful listening, accurate interpretation of what is heard, quick internalization (gestalt formation) of what is heard, then identification of pictures that illustrate what the examiner said or explanation of certain information asked for by the examiner.

Auditory dyslexics cannot score well on these verbal tests. Children like Mary usually comprehend only thirty to forty percent of what they hear the first time. If the examiner is forbidden by standardized test procedures from repeating or rephrasing in simpler terms, Mary is stuck with only partly understood auditory concepts. She is left to guess, say nothing, or panic depending upon her disposition. It is incredibly embarrassing to be an auditory dyslexic. Very little of what the child hears makes sense, especially on standardized tests. Mary almost never gets the point of oral situations as quickly as her peers. She sits isolated inside invisible walls feeling "dumb." Many auditory dyslexics develop cover-up behaviors that greatly irritate adults who do not understand the reason why the child "acts silly" or gives strange or irrelevant responses to oral statements.

An auditory dyslexic is equally handicapped in naming rhyming words, interpreting diacritical markings, applying phonic generalizations, and pronouncing words accurately. Because she does not perceive differences in similar vowel sounds, Mary cannot tell the difference between "big" and "beg," unless she hears the words used in context. An easily observed aspect of her auditory limitation is her garbled pronunciation of familiar words.

For example, Mary is asked to read aloud the following passage from her science book:

> To test for acidity, place one teaspoon of bicarbonate of soda in a beaker. Measure one-fourth cup of vinegar, then pour slowly over the soda. Be sure not to use an aluminum cup.

Because she does not associate sounds and symbols accurately, she reads aloud:

> To test for *a-kye-da-ty,* place one *tee-poon* of *bi-kair-nate* of soda in a *braker. May-zer* one-*for* cup *vigener,* then *pore slow* over the soda. Be sure not to use *alunumum* cup.

This tendency toward garbled speech (echolalia; see Glossary) often embarrasses Mary. She does not understand why others laugh at her tongue twisters.

Auditory dyslexia is difficult to correct because the child is cut off from the fundamental sound-symbol relationships which constitute literacy. It is possible to devise drills and exercises for children like Mary, but this remedial work requires enormous patience on the part of both the teacher and child. As a rule, auditory dyslexics must devise their own sight-memory systems for coping with spelling and related tasks.

Many intelligent dyslexics have mastered common spelling patterns through mnemonic (memory) techniques. For example, Mary has learned to spell "then" and "when" correctly by remembering: *"Then* is *hen* with *t* in front; *when* is *hen* with *w* in front."* Generally, the most effective teaching procedure for auditory dyslexia involves "word families," or spelling patterns. When similar configurations are structured in groups, Mary can memorize enough associations to satisfy ordinary curriculum requirements.

Dysgraphia

A third type of dyslexia is the inability to coordinate hand and arm muscles to write legibly. Many bright dyslexic children have been seriously misjudged because their teachers could not read their written responses. The work of extremely dysgraphic children actually resembles "chicken scratching," with few recognizable letter or word forms on the page. Often these disabled students fill page after page with scribbling in order to appear busy. Frequently they can read their own writing, although no one else can. It is difficult for such dyslexics to learn to write legibly, although certain handwriting drills can increase the legibility of their work. Usually such students can learn to type, thus acquiring a substitute script through which they can communicate in printed form.

Most cases of dysgraphia involve partially legible handwriting. Such writing is often quite small with many poorly formed letters. Many dysgraphics, however, write large with awkwardly broken letter forms. The most effective teaching attitude is to help the dysgraphic student strive for legibility, not perfection. As with other dyslexics, dysgraphic children cannot cope with pressure and speed. Efforts by teachers to hurry or perfect these children result only in frustration and an increasingly poor self-concept.

Dyslexia in the Classroom

Rarely does a child exhibit only one form of dyslexia. Visual dyslexia is usually accompanied by auditory dyslexia, which complicates the teacher's task. It is essential that these factors be identified because, as a rule, only one disability can be corrected at a time. An important characteristic of dyslexia is that multiple stimuli tend to cancel each other out. This means that most dyslexic children cannot master written symbols at the same time they are drilling on phonics. Corrective teaching must provide clearly structured sequences which involve one basic skill at a time. By moving carefully from one skill to another, most dyslexics can overcome many of their limitations within a regular classroom.

If dyslexia is to be corrected, it must be identified early in a child's school experience. Clinical experience shows that time is a critical factor in solving perceptual disabilities. Follow-up studies of dyslexic students indicate a rather somber prognosis.[1] If dyslexia is diagnosed before the child enters Grade Three, there is approximately an eighty percent chance that the child can overcome his confusion with language symbols. If the condition is not diagnosed until Grade Five, there is a forty percent chance of correcting the handicap. For dyslexics who reach Grade Seven before treatment, there is only about five percent chance for sufficient correction to enable the student to reach independent grade level proficiencies in encoding and decoding. Obviously the hopes for successful remediation of adult dyslexics are small.

As the following chapters illustrate, it is not only possible but also feasible for classroom teachers to discover the three faces of dyslexia among their pupils. When the symptoms are recognized early, much can be done within the regular classroom structure to correct these handicaps in children.

References for Further Reading

1. Adams, R. B. "Dyslexia: A Discussion of Its Definition." *Journal of Learning Disabilities* 2 (December 1969): 618-633.

2. Bannatyne, Alex. "Mirror Images and Reversals." *Academic Therapy* 8 (Fall 1972): 87-92.

3. Blom, G. E., and Jones, A. "Bases of Classification of Reading Disorders." *Reading Forum: NINDS* Monograph no. 11, National Institute of Neurological Diseases and Stroke. Washington, D.C.: U.S. Department of Health, Education, and Welfare (1971): 11-30.

4. Brewer, William. "Dyslexia: Neurological and Genetic Etiology." *Reading Forum: NINDS* Monograph no. 11, National Institute of Neurological Diseases and Stroke. Washington, D.C.: U.S. Department of Health, Education, and Welfare, 1971, pp. 47-54.

5. Bryan, Tanis H. "Peer Popularity of Learning Disabled Children." *Journal of Learning Disabilities* 7 (December 1974): 621-625.

---

[1] This estimate is based on unpublished research by the staff of Clinical Services in Reading, Central State University, Edmond, Oklahoma (1968–1971).

6. Carner, R. L. "The Adult Dyslexic—Dilemma and Challenge." *Reading Disability and Perception.* Newark, Delaware: International Reading Association, Proceedings of the 13th Annual Convention, vol. 13, part 3 (1969): 22-28.

7. Chalfant, James C., and King, Frank S. "An Approach to Operationalizing the Definition of Learning Disabilities." *Journal of Learning Disabilities* 9 (April 1976): 228-243.

8. Clarke, Louise. *Can't Read, Can't Write, Can't Talk Too Good Either: How to Recognize and Overcome Dyslexia in Your Child.* New York: Walker and Company, 1973.

9. Clements, Sam D. "Minimal Brain Dysfunction in Children." *Children with Learning Problems.* Edited by Selma G. Sapir and Ann C. Nitzburg, pp. 159-172. New York: Brunner/Mazel, Publishers, 1973.

10. Critcheley, Macdonald. "Developmental Dyslexia as a Specific Cognitive Disorder." *Cognitive Studies: Deficits In Cognition.* Edited by Jerome Hellmuth. vol. 2, pp. 47-52. New York: Brunner/Mazel, Publishers, 1971.

11. Denckla, Martha B. "Clinical Syndromes in Learning Disabilities: The Case for Splitting Versus 'Lumping.'" *Journal of Learning Disabilities* 5 (August/September 1972): 401-406.

12. deQuiros, Julio B. "Significance of Some Therapies on Posture and Learning." *Academic Therapy II* (Spring 1976): 261-270.

13. De Hirsch, Katrina. "Specific Dyslexia or Strephosymbolia." *Children with Reading Problems.* Edited by Gladys Natchez. pp. 97-113. New York: Basic Books, 1968.

14. Di Leo, J. H. "Early Identification of Minimal Cerebral Dysfunction." *Academic Therapy Quarterly* 5 (Spring 1970): 187-203.

15. Edwards, R. P., *et al.* "Academic Achievement and Minimal Brain Dysfunction." *Journal of Learning Disabilities* 4 (March 1971): 134-138.

16. Gaston, E. B., and Jones, A. W. "Bases of Classification of Reading Disorders." *Journal of Learning Disabilities* 3 (December 1970): 606-617.

17. Gibson, Eleanor J., and Levin, Harry. *The Psychology of Reading.* Cambridge, Massachusetts: The M.I.T. Press, 1975. pp. 485-487.

18. Gross, Mortimer B., and Wilson, William C. *Minimal Brain Dysfunction.* New York: Brunner/Mazel, Publishers, 1974.

19. Howards, Melvin. "An Interpretation of Dyslexia—An Educator's Viewpoint." *Reading Disability and Perception.* Newark, Delaware: International Reading Association, Proceedings of the 13th Annual Convention, vol. 13, part 3 (1969): 8-15.

20. Isom, J. B. "An Interpretation of Dyslexia—A Medical Viewpoint." *Reading Disability and Perception.* Newark, Delaware: International Reading

Association, Proceedings of the 13th Annual Convention, 13 (1969): 8-15.

21. Kagan, Jerome. "Dyslexia and Its Remediation." *Reading Forum: NINDS* Monograph no. 11, National Institute of Neurological Diseases and Stroke. Washington, D.C.: U.S. Department of Health, Education, and Welfare, 1971, pp. 55-64.

22. Klasen, Edith. *The Syndrome of Specific Dyslexia.* Baltimore: University Park Press, 1972.

23. Klees, Marianne, and Lebrun, Ariane. "Analysis of the Figurative and Operative Processes of Thought of Forty Dyslexic Children." *Journal of Learning Disabilities* 5 (August/September 1972): 389-396.

24. Knobloch, Hilda, and Pasamanick, Benjamin. *Developmental Diagnosis: The Evaluation and Management of Normal and Abnormal Neuropsychologic Development in Infancy and Early Childhood.* 3d ed. New York: Harper and Row, 1974.

25. Koppitz, Elizabeth M. *Children with Learning Disabilities: A Five Year Follow-up Study.* New York: Grune & Stratton, 1971.

26. Lockavitch, Joseph F. "Of Course I'm Not Stupid . . . . I Just Don't Know My Right from My Left." *Academic Therapy Publications* 10 (Winter 1974-75): 159-165.

27. McClurg, W. H. "Dyslexia: Early Identification and Treatment in the Schools." *Journal of Learning Disabilities* 3 (April 1970): 232-233.

28. McGuire, M. L. "Dyslexia: A Reading Specialist's Opinion." *Journal of Learning Disabilities* 3 (July, 1970): 232-233.

29. Meier, John H. "Prevalence and Characteristics of Learning Disabilities Found in Second Grade Children." *Journal of Learning Disabilities* 4 (January 1971): 1-16.

30. Money, John. "On Learning and Not Learning to Read." *The Disabled Reader: Education of the Dyslexic Child.* Edited by John Money, pp. 21-40. Baltimore: The Johns Hopkins Press, 1966.

31. Orton, Samuel. "An Impediment to Learning to Read—A Neurological Explanation of Reading Disability." *Children with Reading Problems.* Edited by Gladys Natchez, pp. 89-96. New York: Basic Books, 1968.

32. Rice, Donald. "Learning Disabilities: An Investigation in Two Parts—Part II: Implications for School Curriculum and Program Planning." *Journal of Learning Disabilities* 3 (April 1970): 193-199.

33. Rossi, Albert O. "Genetics of Higher Level Disorders." *Journal of Learning Disabilities* 3 (August 1970): 386-390.

34. _____. "Genetics of Learning Disabilities." *Journal of Learning Disabilities* 5 (October 1972): 489-496.

35. Schleichkorn, Jacob. "The Teacher and Recognition of Problems in Children." *Journal of Learning Disabilities* 5 (October 1972): 501-502.

36. Serio, Martha. "Know the Child to Teach the Child: A Checklist." *Academic Therapy Quarterly* 5 (Spring 1970): 222-227.

37. Silver, Larry B. "A Proposed View on the Etiology of the Neurological Learning Disability Syndrome." *Journal of Learning Disabilities* 4 (March 1971): 123-133.

38. _____. "Familial Patterns in Children with Neurologically-Based Learning Disabilities." *Journal of Learning Disabilities* 4 (August/September 1971): 349-358.

39. Slingerland, B. H. "Early Identification of Preschool Children Who Might Fail." *Academic Therapy Quarterly* 6 (Spring 1969): 245-252.

40. Smith, B. K. "Dilemma of a Dyslexic Man." Austin, Texas: The Hogg Foundation for Mental Health, The University of Texas, 1969.

41. Strother, C. R. "Minimal Cerebral Dysfunction: An Historical Overview." *Children with Learning Problems.* Edited by Selma G. Sapir and Ann C. Nitzburg, pp. 173-186. New York: Brunner/Mazel Publishers, 1973.

42. Templeton, A. B., *et al. Reading Disorders in the United States: Report of the Secretary's (HEW) National Advisory Committee on Dyslexia and Reading Disorders.* Washington, D.C.: United States Government Printing Office, 1969.

43. Thompson, Lloyd J. "Language Disabilities in Men of Eminence." *Journal of Learning Disabilities* 4 (January 1971): 34-35.

44. Thompson, Lloyd J. "Learning Disabilities: An Overview." *American Journal of Psychiatry* 130 (April 1973) 393-399.

45. Vernon, M. D. "Specific Dyslexia." In *Children with Reading Problems.* Edited by Gladys Natchez, pp. 114-121. New York: Basic Books, 1968.

46. Vogel, Susan Ann. *Syntatic Abilities in Normal and Dyslexic Children.* Baltimore: University Park Press, 1975.

47. Wagner, R. F. "Symbolization Deficits in Dyslexic Conditions." *Academic Therapy Quarterly* 6 (Summer 1971): 359-365.

48. Weil, Annemarie P. "Children with Minimal Brain Dysfunction: Diagnostic, Dynamic, and Therapeutic Considerations." *Children with Learning Problems.* Edited by Selma G. Sapir and Ann C. Nitzburg, pp. 551-568. New York: Brunner/Mazel Publishers, 1973.

49. Wendes, Paul H. *Minimal Brain Dysfunction in Children.* New York: Wiley-Interscience, 1971.

chapter 2

Visual Dyslexia in the Classroom

AS DESCRIBED IN CHAPTER 1, VISUAL DYSLEXIA REFERS TO THE IN-ability to interpret printed symbols accurately. Although this inhibition is somewhat mysterious, it can be identified by teachers who are alert to its symptoms. As far as classroom performance is concerned, visual dyslexia is basically the failure to keep symbols in correct order. Whether the handicapped child is scanning words or trying to recall items in sequence, the visual dyslexic cannot accurately follow the sequential order he encounters in encoded language (2, 13, 15, 16, 18, 20).

Visual Dyslexia Syndrome

There is no single behavior characteristic which establishes dyslexia. All children manifest faulty perception in various stages of maturation. Before visual dyslexia can be confirmed, a set, or syndrome, of be-haviors must be identified. Only when an unmistakable cluster of per-ceptual disabilities is diagnosed can a teacher safely conclude that a child is dyslexic.

Confusion with Sequence

The underlying flaw in visual dyslexia is the child's inability to compre-hend order or sequence. Few classroom teachers fully realize how much of the school day is geared to following this model:

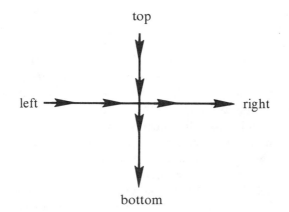

All reading, except for special instances in certain content areas, must be done left-to-right from the top to the bottom of the column or page. This principle is so commonly taken for granted that almost no reminders are made by teachers above the primary grades. It is assumed that any child who reads will automatically do so within this framework. Unfortunately, this is not so for dyslexics.

The dyslexic orientation is the opposite, or partly so. The dyslexic tendency is "mirror image," meaning that the student's nature is to process symbols backwards (right-to-left and bottom-to-top). In fact, one of the developmental milestones we look for in kindergarten pupils is the point at which they "turn it over" and begin to conform to the standard directionality of school materials. Approximately eighty percent of the student population achieves this standard left-to-right, top-to-bottom orientation successfully, although late maturing children may not do so until second or third grade. The remaining twenty percent never fully achieve this standard orientation. Most of them are dyslexic.

Unfortunately for Mike, his primary teachers did not understand his difficulty with directionality. When the reading teacher introduced the letter d, she assumed that all of her pupils perceived it left-to-right (ball first, then the stick) and top-to-bottom (stick pointing up from the ball). Mike was completely unaware of his different orientation. He perceived the letter d right-to-left (stick first, then the ball) and bottom-to-top (stick below the ball). What the teacher perceived as d, Mike perceived as p. Several critical symbols are thus misperceived by dyslexic learners: d—b—p—q M—W u—n 7—L 6—9 h—y. When dyslexics only partly rotate symbols, they often confuse N—Z and 3—M—W.

The unfortunate consequence is that Mike is constantly told he is wrong. Unless someone explains how his perception differs, he enters the reading and writing process with no idea that he is heading the wrong direction up a very busy street. This is why he constantly collides with on-coming traffic. His teachers and most of his peers are proceeding in one direction while he travels the opposite or partly opposite way. So long as this situation is not recognized and understood, there is no way he can master the symbol system without constant conflict and the put-down of always being wrong.

Generally, this disability functions whenever the dyslexic tries to deal with time, arrangement, or relationships of entities along a continuum. For example, instead of recalling an orderly progression of experiences in relation to time, Mike's memory stock of early childhood is a jumbled collection of events which do not fall into an orderly time sequence. In his perception of time, a broken arm of two months ago happened right after he badly bruised his elbow when he was three. Grandmother's death five years ago seems like last month to Mike.

Most children have a confused memory of their early years, but those with normal receptive processes learn to view their experiences in an ordered sequence as they mature. Visual dyslexics do not. Since mastery of language symbols depends upon comprehension of sequence and interrelatedness of symbols, this perceptual limitation is the greatest obstacle facing the visual dyslexic in today's curriculum.

Confusion with sequence is a definite factor in Mike's ability to accept responsibility. Because of his general frustration with order and sequence, he is almost constantly in conflict with adult demands. At home his parents have given him the following responsibilities to be done each weekday morning: 1. Make bed before breakfast. 2. Brush teeth after breakfast. 3. Feed and water pets before catching school bus. 4. Take all homework back to school for day's classwork.

In the afternoon Mike faces another set of responsibilities: 1. Empty trash baskets on Monday, Wednesday, and Friday. 2. Feed and water pets every afternoon. 3. Attend Cub Scouts on Tuesday afternoon. 4. Sweep garage on Saturday. 5. Read Sunday school lesson before bedtime on Saturday. 6. Pick up toys and tools from yard before noon on Saturday. 7. Bathe dog either Saturday or Sunday afternoon. 8. Be bathed and ready for bed by 9:00 o'clock each night.

These adult expectations have never been put into outline form or in tangible chronological sequence for Mike. His parents have dictated these routines orally, assuming that he perceives time and sequence as clearly as they do. Mike's dyslexic tendencies to scramble the order of things, however, leaves him with an unstructured mass of responsibilities. In spite of his intentions to obey his parents, he finds himself confused and frustrated. As his chores remain undone, adults conclude that the boy is lazy, stubborn, insubordinate, or forgetful. In reality, Mike is filled with dread and self-defeat. He has no way to communicate his dilemma to the adults who are obviously displeased with him. His unfinished chores generate family friction and almost constant misery for the child. After this kind of situation has gone uncorrected for several years, Mike has indeed become insubordinate and hostile. By the time he enters middle school he is convinced that he is worthless and incapable of success.

Similar frustration occurs in the classroom between uninformed teachers and confused children like Mike. With so many pupils to care for, the teacher quite naturally assumes that her instructions to Group A have been clear. As she turns to Group B, she is annoyed to see Mike not following her directions. Again the dyslexic child has failed in his relationships with the adult world. Since he cannot communicate his confusion to the teacher, she usually rejects him as being lazy, careless, or insubordinate. Thus the teacher has unwittingly set the stage for misbehavior and unhappiness. Mike's failure to follow class instructions is due to perceptual difficulty in comprehending sequence, not wilfull disobedience.

In the classroom an alert teacher can identify confusion with sequence as pupils work with tasks involving series. For example, dyslexic children like Mike are usually fluent in oral reporting and conversation. Casual listeners are generally well impressed by his stock of information and concepts gleaned through listening and observation. There is, however, a noticeable flaw in his oral performance. He has difficulty recalling the correct sequence of details.

Many visual dyslexics cannot remember the day, month, and year of their birth. The teacher can check for this tendency through informal conversation in the room. Although he may know reams of statistics about his favorite ball team, Mike will usually stumble when asked to tell his full birth date.

He also has difficulty naming the days of the week and the months of the year. When asked to write or recite this rote information, he keeps track by tapping his fingers, mumbling a rhyme, or singing a song. An interesting earmark of visual dyslexia is Mike's tendency to skip October when reciting the months, probably because October does not rhyme with September, November, and December. In arithmetic, Mike will have enormous problems learning the multiplication tables, long division, interrelationships between decimals/fractions/percent, mental computation involving money and measurement, and myriad other number skills.

The following examples from the Jordan Written Screening Test for Specific Reading Disability (see Appendix B) illustrate this problem with familiar items in sequence. The teacher not only gains a quick insight into sequence failure, but she also begins to see evidence of dysgraphia and auditory dyslexia, if these disabilities exist.

Another informal estimate of Mike's comprehension of sequence is to ask him to repeat a series of numbers. For example, he listens as the teacher says "6–8–7–9–2." Then the teacher observes his efforts to repeat the numbers in the same sequence. Visual dyslexics usually fail in this kind of serial task. Or Mike might listen to a sentence and then repeat it verbatim: "Three men raced down the hill to their

1. Write the Alphabet

a B C D E F G h l J K l m n o p Q R S T U V W x y z

2. Write your Birthday (month, day, and year)

fono 18   5 8

3. Write the Days of the Week

Sun. Mun. Tun. Wes. Thor. Frl Sat

4. Write the Months of the Year

Jon, Frab Mer, april, may, June, Jaly, Avgst, Sep, Oct, nov, Dec, boat in the river" (see Appendix B, Items 16 and 17 on the Jordan Written Screening Test). It is characteristic of dyslexics to omit complete phrases or to substitute different words. Frequently they lose the theme of the sentence entirely.

Faulty Reading Comprehension

Faulty perception of sequence is a major reason for Mike's poor performance on reading comprehension tests. Although a majority of students exhibit inferior comprehension to some degree, visual dyslexics are especially susceptible to faulty retention of information presented in sequence.

Conservation of Form. The pioneering work of Bärbel Inhelder and Jean Piaget has given us a simple yet profound framework within which we may understand the growth of logic in children (3, 6, 12, 14). Their term "conservation of form" is especially helpful in understanding the dyslexic learning dilemma. Conservation of visual form refers to the ability to see specific forms (letters, numerals, words, or shapes), then hold those images intact after the model is taken away. The act of reading could be described in this way. As the reader sees visual forms on the printed page, his memory systems are expected to make lasting impressions which the reader uses later after he has put the book aside or after his eyes have left a particular point of focus. Visual dyslexics cannot do this perceptual act successfully. Students like Mike do not conserve the form. Once the model is no longer in view the mental image (gestalt) is lost, or parts of it are lost. The dyslexic reader conserves only bits and pieces of the whole model he has seen. In addition to conserving only part of the whole, he rotates or reverses or scrambles the sequence of the parts. Severely dyslexic students cannot conserve form for more than a few seconds (very short-term memory). The moment their eyes move away from single words or parts of words, the mental image is lost or scrambled. Reading comprehension is especially difficult and tedious. Sometimes it is impossible to achieve.

Reversibility. Conservation of form also involves the ability to change form (transformation). In changing a statement into a question, for example, the reader must hold the author's meaning (conserve the form) well enough to restructure the order of the words. Teachers of language arts can testify to how difficult it is to teach dyslexics this operation in building variations of sentences. Reversibility is at the heart of arithmetic computation, especially when children must deal with such linear form as ___ + 5 = 9. Unless a child can transform this visual pattern into

$$\begin{array}{r} 5 \\ + \\ \hline 9 \end{array}$$

he will be totally confused by modern math.

As he reads or listens, Mike's receptive processes do not maintain a consistent intake of information. Just as he does not perceive an orderly sequence of time, neither does he comprehend the organization of an author's prose. When asked specific recall questions about his silent reading, Mike cannot retrieve enough organized information to respond as most teachers expect. This chronic failure to comprehend creates an aversion to reading early in the visual dyslexic's school experience.

This handicap is particularly punitive when Mike is asked to draw inferences or to arrive at conclusions quickly. Standardized reading tests which require the child to read paragraphs and then answer questions within a strict time limitation are almost impossible tasks for dyslexics. When given ample time, pupils like Mike can often arrive at satisfactory answers through trial and error or through the process of eliminating irrelevant answers. But timed pressure only increases the erratic comprehension patterns which plague visual dyslexics even under the most relaxed study conditions.

Teachers universally bewail Mike's tendency to "guess" on pressure tests. Skipping down the page, marking items at random, or refusing to check back over his work for errors are perfectly reasonable responses, however, in view of his perceptual handicap. By the time he has experienced three or more years of failure to comprehend what he reads, there is actually little else for Mike to do but guess, especially when told that no consideration will be made for his slow pace, the only speed at which he can succeed.

Difficulty with the Alphabet

Of major concern to primary teachers is the visual dyslexic's inability to cope with the alphabet. The unstructured way in which the alphabet is introduced to primary pupils is largely to blame for uncorrected visual dyslexia. For half a century elementary teachers have studiously avoided rote learning of the alphabet by beginner children. Clinicians have known for years that beginners have been learning the alphabetic sequence on their own, usually from charts displayed in primary classrooms. Educators, however, have generally discouraged direct teaching of the alphabetic sequence before Grade Two.

This unstructured approach has posed no problem for most children. Pupils with normal perception usually acquire knowledge of the alphabet as they need it, thus vindicating professors who advise teachers to avoid rote learning. However well meaning this philosophy may be, it has denied dyslexic children the only learning context in which they can succeed, that of a structured, direct encounter with specifics. Since the visual dyslexic's principal weakness is faulty perception of sequence, having little or no sequence to follow proves disastrous when he is confronted with symbol systems. Had Mike been well grounded in alphabetic sequence at the very beginning of his school experience, he could have coped with beginning reading tasks more successfully.

A simple technique for determining a child's perception of the alphabet is for the teacher to watch him write it on ruled paper. Any dyslexic tendencies will quickly become apparent. Children with normal perception usually write the alphabet in sequence without hesitation. Visual dyslexics cannot.

When asked to write the alphabet, Mike will often stall, asking whether he should print or "write cursy." When told that it does not matter, he may want to know if he should use big or little letters. Dyslexic children seldom comprehend the terms "capital" and "lowercase." Next Mike may ask whether he should go across or down the page. When finally at work, he will reach a stalling point, often at letter M. Whenever he bogs down, he goes back to A and whispers the letters one by one, trying to remember the whole sequence. Occasionally he will hum the alphabet song to himself. The observer can easily note the dyslexic's problem of synchronizing speech with writing. Mike's voice will usually be ahead of his eyes or finger. Consequently, reviewing his written work still does not help him identify errors.

Mike is very slow as he writes or prints the alphabet. The letters m, n, p, u, and v are often in scrambled positions. In addition to this serial problem, he confuses similar letters, such as b–d–p–q r–h–u–n h–p–y t–f–j M–W N–Z r–s v–w–k–y–x and o–e–c.

As he writes, Mike makes certain letters with backward hand motions. He frequently forms circular components of letters with a clockwise motion, as well as marking from the bottom upward when writing t, f, p, g, b, or d. Unless the teacher is carefully observing his work, she might not be aware of this backward motion, an earmark of dyslexia.

It is common for the visual dyslexic to mix capital and lowercase letters when writing the alphabet, as well as mixing manuscript and cursive styles. Mike's reasons for this inconsistent writing are actually quite practical. Because he has not been taught the sequence of the alphabet, thereby never having encountered the letters in relation to each other in a continuum, he has devised his own system for identifying certain letter forms. B and D are stable in his perception, although they may be written backwards, while b is too easily confused with d, p, or q. So long as he continues to deal with isolated letters in manuscript style, there is no dependable structure to which Mike can anchor his perceptions of the alphabet.

The following handwriting specimens illustrate these dyslexic tendencies. It is unfortunate that well-meaning adults misinterpret such handicapped work as the mark of inferior intellect or "laziness."

Jeff

Age: 6 years, 7 months
Grade: 1.8
IQ: 133 Stanford-Binet

a B c d e f G H i l k l m n o p
o q s t y w x s

Paul

Age: 7 years, 3 months
Grade: 2.2
IQ: 135

Lewis

Age: 14 years, 7 months
Grade: 8.8
IQ: 109

b → J
x → +
e → c
r → P
m → w
7 → 7 f

b → P
d → q
h → n
f → A
6 → E
q → q

Lewis
Age: 14 years, 7 months
Grade: 8.8
IQ: 109 Stanford-Binet

A B C D E F G H

I K L M N o p q u R s T

W y z

Jim
Age: 26 years, 4 months
Grade: College sophomore
IQ: 103 WAIS

A B C D E F g H & g K L m n o p q R

s u g u v w x y z

Lesli
female Age: 6 years, 7 months
Grade: 1.6
IQ: 114 Stanford-Binet

A B C P F G H i J K L W h O P Q

r t y V M x y s

Jim
Age: 7 years, 6 months
Grade: 2.8
IQ: 113 WISC

A a B d C c D b E e f g h i J K L n m o p Q

r S t u v x y x

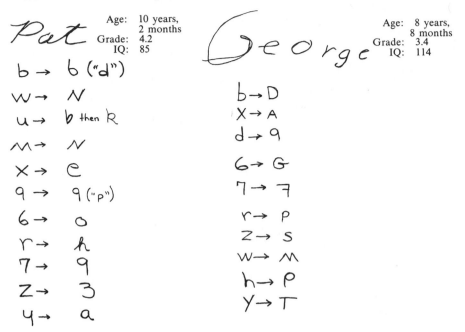

For further insight into a child's perception, the teacher traces symbols on the pupil's back. Then the child writes what he "saw" on the chalkboard. The pupil may write in cursive style when the teacher has traced in manuscript. No issue should be made of this, however. The purpose of tracing on the back is to identify the child's immediate perception of (reaction to) symbols, not to test his recognition of writing style.

The previous specimens illustrate the insights which this test can yield. In each case the symbols traced by the teacher are in the left column with the pupil responses on the right.

Reversal of Symbols

An earmark of dyslexia is the child's confusion as to the direction certain symbols should face. This faulty perception causes the pupil to write or read symbols backwards, upside down, or partially rotated. This tendency is illustrated in the following writing specimen. As described earlier in the chapter, dyslexics generally use capital B and D as a means of distinguishing between these similar letter forms. The following specimen also illustrates dysgraphia (see Chapter 4).

Dictated by Teacher	Dyslexic Responses
bad	*Bab*
bag	*Bag*
ball	*Ball*
bed	*Bed*
bell	*Bell*
big	*Big*
bill	*Bill*
body	*Boby*
bug	*Bug*
dad	*Dab*
did	*Did*
dog	*Dog*
doll	*Doll*

Oral Reading

The tendency to reverse or rotate symbols is a handicap in reading printed materials. Often dyslexics read whole words in reverse. Sometimes only certain kinds of syllables are reversed within words. Initial letters, especially lowercase b, d, p, q, h, r, m, w, and u, are frequently perceived upside down or backwards, causing the reader to mistake many words for others that are similar. This results in nonsense, forcing the dyslexic reader to study the context of the material to find his mistaken word recognition. Dyslexics usually are able to learn techniques of self-correction when their patterns of faulty perception are pointed out to them.

The teacher can detect this tendency by listening as her pupils read aloud from printed materials. Within a few minutes she can identify children with reversal habits. A simple instrument for classroom use is the JOST—Jordan Oral Screening Test (see Appendix A). As the child reads aloud, the teacher makes rapid notes of errors. Careful observation reveals any dyslexic patterns in the pupil's handling of word elements.

The following oral reading errors often indicate dyslexia:

1. Reversal of Beginning Letters
   "bark" for dark   "dump" for bump
2. Transposition of Blends and Digraphs
   "preform" for perform   "there" for three
   "star" for stream   "porfit" for profit
3. Substitution of One Similar Letter for Another
   "sleep" for sheep   "come" for came
4. Transposition of Letters within Words
   "magilant" for malignant   "macilous" for malicious
5. Reversal of Whole Words
   "on" for no   "saw" for was   "but" for tub
6. Failure to Perceive Minimal Cues
   "house" for horse   "with" for wish
   "butter" for better   "hungry" for hunger
   This includes habitual failure to perceive punctuation cues.
7. Omission of Endings
   "ever" for every   "her" for here   "happen" for happened
8. Telescoping
   "standarize" for standardize   "consently" for consequently
   "sudly" for suddenly
9. Perseveration
   "hopenen" for hope   "sudendely" for suddenly
   "farmerer" for farmer

Dyslexia is suspected only when several of these symptoms exist in the child's oral reading. Teachers must be careful to distinguish between faulty vision and dyslexia (see Chapter 8).

Errors in Copying

An especially difficult task for dyslexics is copying information from the chalkboard or from a projection screen. This involves conservation of form, also called vision-to-motor transfer. The child must see the forms clearly, hold them intact (conserve) as he moves his focus to the writing space, translate what he saw into specific motor movements (fine motor control), space it properly on the writing paper (figure/ground control), and end up with a legible facsimile of what was on the chalkboard or in the text from which he was copying. Busy teachers often forget what a complex task copying really is. It is a monumental task for dyslexics who do not conserve form without enormous concentration and effort. The advent of visual aids has increased the pressure on many students to take notes while the teacher lectures with an overhead projector. The basic problems with symbol confusion handicap a visual dyslexic in such a task setting. His slow work rate, confusion with symbols, and frustration with keeping items in correct sequence combine to make copying from a distance a hazardous undertaking (8).

The teacher can rather easily identify which of her pupils is handicapped by far-point copying. A neatly lettered or handwritten paragraph can be put on the chalkboard or large chart. Each pupil is asked to copy the paragraph from across the room. As the children work at copying, the teacher watches for these tendencies:

1. Losing place on chart
2. Erasing frequently
3. Overprinting to correct mistakes on paper
4. Misspelling on paper
5. Failing to observe capital letters
6. Failing to observe punctuation cues
7. Failing to space properly on paper
8. Reversing letters
9. Reversing whole words
10. Working unusually slowly

These flaws in performance can also be caused by certain defects of vision (see Chapter 8). The teacher must be careful not to mistake dyslexic confusion of sequence with specific vision defects.

The following example of copying errors illustrates the dyslexic difficulty with far-point copying. The story is from the JWST—Jordan Written Screening Test for Specific Reading Disabilities (see Appendix B).

Bob and Dan

Bob and Dan saw Sam Watts on the dock. The three men stopped.
"See the big ship?" asked Sam.
"Sure did," Dan and Bob said.
"Must be a mile long."
Bob and Dan saw Sam was in a hurry. "Got to run," Sam said.
"See you."
"Sure," said Bob and Dan. "See you, Sam."

Bob and Don

Bob and Don saw Sam Watts on the dock. The three men stopped. See the big ship?" asked Son. Sure did" Dan and Bob said. "Must be a mile long." Bob and Don saw Son was in a hurry. "Got to run." Sam said. See you." "Sure," said Bob. "See you, Son"

Errors in Spelling

There is a unique pattern of spelling error which distinguishes visual dyslexia from auditory dyslexia. Because the primary disability is not being able to handle items in sequence, the visual dyslexic cannot recall a clear mental image of whole word forms. Usually the student is able to identify most of the sound units which make up specific words, but the letters will be in scrambled order when he writes the word. The visual dyslexic can identify the sound elements in common words. His problem is not being able to record them in correct sequence.

The following errors illustrate visual dyslexia in spelling from memory. The teacher must keep in mind that this pattern may also be found in other forms of learning disability.

Word in Mike's mind	His written response
rode	roed
ate	aet
goes	gose
heaven	haveen
marriage	mirarage

Checklist of Visual Dyslexia Symptoms

Through extensive work with children and classroom teachers, the author has devised the following informal checklist for identifying visual dyslexia. It is important that teachers withhold judgment until a definite syndrome of dyslexic symptoms has been identified in a pupil's behavior. If a significant cluster of perceptual errors appears as the teacher studies a child's behavior, then it is generally safe to conclude that visual dyslexia exists in the pupil's perceptual processes. However, the checklists in Chapter 8 must also be considered so that certain other disabilities are not mistaken for dyslexia.

_____Confusion with Sequence

   _____has poor concept of time
   _____has poor concept of chronological order of events
   _____cannot give day, month, and year of birth
   _____cannot repeat months of year
   _____cannot repeat days of week
   _____cannot remember multiplication tables

_____Difficulty Following Directions

   _____cannot remember daily routines at home
   _____cannot follow teacher's directions in classroom
   _____cannot comprehend instructions when given to a group; needs individual explanations
   _____needs constant reminding of what to do

_____Faulty Oral Language

   is fluent at telling stories or giving oral reports
   _____discusses information from nonreading sources
   has difficulty with correct sequence of events

_____Faulty Reading Comprehension

   _____fails to identify main ideas
   _____tells story events out of sequence
   _____loses meaning of sentences or paragraphs before reaching the end
   _____fails to draw inferences from what has been read
   _____has difficulty recalling details when answering comprehensive questions

_____Slow Work Rate

   _____seldom finishes timed exercises
   _____easily frustrated when pressured for speed
   _____work pace considerably slower than classmates
   _____can do satisfactory work if given ample time and help

_____will not use full time allowance on timed tests; guesses, marking items at random

_____Difficulty with Alphabet

_____does not know alphabet in correct sequence
_____omits certain letters from alphabetic sequence
_____mixes capital and lowercase letters
_____mixes manuscript and cursive styles
_____confuses similar letters
_____makes certain letters backward, upside down
_____sings alphabet song or repeats rhyme to check sequence
_____is not able to synchronize voice, finger, and eyes while checking work

_____Confusion with Symbols

_____demonstrates poor perception when symbols are traced on back

_____perceives symbols upside down
_____perceives symbols backward
_____distorts shapes of symbols
_____rotates positions of symbols
_____writes with capital B and D
_____confuses certain symbols in reading, writing, and arithmetic
_____cannot conserve form in copy work

_____b – d – p – q		_____h – n
_____h – y		_____m – w
_____r – n		_____l – i
_____r – c – s		_____n – u
_____f – t		_____N – Z
_____3 – E		_____6 – 9
		_____ + × , – ÷

_____Errors in Oral Reading

_____reverses whole words
_____reverses beginning letters
_____transposes l and r in consonant blends
_____substitutes similar letters or words
_____transposes letters inside words
_____fails to perceive minimal cues in words
_____fails to perceive minimal cues in punctuation
_____omits endings
_____telescopes (leaves out letters or syllables)
_____perseverates (adds extra letters or syllables)

_____Errors in Spelling

    _____transposes silent letters within words
    _____does not recall correct order of letters
    _____misplaces silent e   .

_____Errors in Arithmetic

    _____reverses processes while computing
    _____carries or borrows wrong digit
    _____cannot organize facts in story problems

_____Errors in Copying

    _____loses place on board (far point)
    _____misspells on paper
    _____fails to observe capital letters
    _____fails to observe punctuation cues
    _____fails to space properly
    _____erases frequently
    _____overprints to correct mistakes
    _____reverses letters
    _____reverses whole words
    _____telescopes
    _____perseverates
    _____works unusually slowly
    _____seeks to terminate to avoid copying tasks

References for Further Reading

1. Baker, Georgia P., and Raskin, Larry M. "Sensory Integration in the Learning Disabled." *Journal of Learning Disabilities* 6 (December 1973): 645-649.

2. Bannatyne, A. D., and Wichiarajote, Penny. "Relationships between Written Spelling, Motor Functioning, and Sequencing Skills." *Journal of Learning Disabilities* 2 (January 1969): 4-16.

3. Bruner, Jerome S. *The Process of Education.* New York: Vintage Books, 1960.

4. Early, George H. "Low-Level Functional Deficits in Learning-Disabled Children," *Academic Therapy Quarterly* 8 (Winter 1972-73): 231-234.

5. Forrest, Elliott B. "The Visual Auditory-Verbal Program." *Journal of Learning Disabilities* 5 (March 1972): 136-144.

6. Friedland, Seymour J., and Meisels, Samuel J. "An Application of the Piagetian Model to Perceptual Handicaps." *Journal of Learning Disabilities* 8 (January 1975): 20-24.

7. Frostig, Marianne. "Visual Perception, Integrative Functions, and Academic Learning." *Journal of Learning Disabilities* 5 (January 1972): 1-15.

8. Goldberg, H. K., and Arnott, William. "Ocular Motility in Learning Disabilities." *Journal of Learning Disabilities* 3 (March 1970): 160-162.

9. Guthrie, John T., and Goldberg, Herman K. "Visual Sequential Memory in Reading Disability." *Journal of Learning Disability* 5 (January 1972): 41-46.

10. Hammill, D. D. "Evaluating Children for Instructional Purposes." *Academic Therapy Quarterly* 6 (Summer 1971): 341-353.

11. Hyman, Joan, and Cohen, S. Alan. "The Effect of Verticality as a Stimulus Property on the Letter Discrimination of Young Children." *Journal of Learning Disabilities* 8 (February 1975): 98-107.

12. Inhelder, Bärbel, and Piaget, Jean. *The Early Growth of Logic in The Child.* New York: Harper and Row, Publishers, 1974.

13. Johnson, Doris J., and Myklebust, Helmer R. *Learning Disabilities: Educational Principles and Practices.* New York: Grune and Stratton, 1967.

14. Kershner, John R. "Conservation of Multiple Space Relations by Children: Effects of Perception and Representation." *Journal of Learning Disabilities* 4 (June/July 1971): 316-321.

15. Kidd, J. W. "The Discriminatory Repertoire—The Basis of All Learning." *Journal of Learning Disabilities* 3 (October 1970): 531-533.

16. Lawrence, J. R., and Potter, R. E. "Visual Motor Disabilities in Children with Functional Articulation Defects." *Journal of Learning Disabilities* 3 (July 1970): 355-358.

17. McNiff, Shaun A. "Art Activities for Evaluating Visual Memory." *Academic Therapy Quarterly* 11 (Spring 1976): 283-296.

18. Maietta, D. F. "The Role of Cognitive Regulators in Learning-Disabled Teenagers." *Academic Therapy Quarterly* 5 (Spring 1970): 177-186.

19. Mattick, Ilse, and Murphy, L. B. "Cognitive Disturbances in Young Children." *Cognitive Studies: Deficits in Cognition.* Edited by Jerome Hellmuth. vol. 2, pp. 280-323. New York: Brunner/Mazel Publishers, 1971.

20. Raskin, Larry M., and Baker, Georgia P. "Tactual and Visual Integration in the Learning Processes: Research and Implications." *Journal of Learning Disabilities* 8 (February 1975): 108-112.

21. Senf, G. M., and Freundl, P. C. "Memory and Attention Factors in Specific Learning Disabilities." *Journal of Learning Disabilities* 4 (February 1971): 94-106.

22. Tinney, Franklin A. "A Comparison of the KeyMath Diagnostic Arithmetic Test and the California Arithmetic Test Used with Learning Disabled Students." *Journal of Learning Disabilities* 8 (May 1975): 313-315.

chapter 3

Auditory Dyslexia in the Classroom

AN OCCUPATIONAL DREAD OF VOCAL MUSIC TEACHERS IS THE MONOTONE child who "can't carry a tune in a bucket." No matter how much musical drill such a student endures, he never learns to cope with vocal music skills. Fortunately these tone deaf children can be assigned to the stage crew, or asked to hand out programs at the door. Unlike vocal instructors, reading teachers do not have alternatives for handicapped students.

Auditory dyslexia is similar to tone deafness. The disability has little to do with hearing acuity, as many dyslexics exhibit keen hearing abilities outside the classroom. Auditory dyslexia refers to the inability to distinguish separate, or discrete, elements of spoken language. Since the child does not perceive the components of oral language accurately, he is unable to associate speech sounds with traditional spelling symbols or patterns. This disability makes it difficult for the student to write down his thoughts according to traditional standards of usage. Auditory dyslexics usually do not master phonics because they do not comprehend, or perceive, sound-symbol relationships accurately (1, 2, 6, 8, 9).

Auditory Dyslexia Syndrome

When diagnosing this disability, teachers must keep in mind that few students master all of the sound-symbol relationships of American speech. Most of us exhibit certain areas of phonetic weakness. The classroom teacher, however, can learn to identify those students who cannot encode oral language into written form. When attempting to read, the auditory dyslexic fails to recognize that the written forms stand for words he uses fluently in daily speech.

A primary characteristic of auditory dyslexia is the inability to comprehend variations of vowel sounds. Most reading programs emphasize the "long" and "short" sounds of five vowels: a, e, i, o, and u. Although w and y are also added to the vowel category, teachers do not always teach specific sound values for these semivowels. Educators have generally assumed that intelligent children with no obvious speech defects should have no difficulty discriminating the long sounds from short sounds. This is not the case with perceptually impaired students. Auditory dyslexics have great difficulty distinguishing such close word forms as "big" and "beg," or "cat" and "cot," unless the words are used in a meaningful context. For the dyslexic child, subtle distinctions in sound values do not exist.

A similar problem is evident when dyslexic students encounter consonant clusters, also called blends and digraphs. Few auditory dyslexics can identify the separate consonant elements in such clusters as st, sp, gr, or pl. Dyslexics usually can identify the initial letter in familiar words. It is frequently impossible, however, for them to identify the second or third element in clusters such as str, spl, or shr.

It is common for auditory dyslexia to remain undetected during the primary grades, particularly when formal phonics and spelling instruction are postponed until Grade Three. Nearly all beginner pupils stumble in their first encounters with organized reading and writing instruction. When the whole-word, or sight-memory, approach is used in primary grades, teachers can remain unaware that certain pupils are not perceiving discrete sounds and symbols accurately.

Confusion with Words: Alike or Different?

One of the earmarks of auditory dyslexia is the student's inability to tell whether words are the same, or whether they are different. Mary is a typical child handicapped by auditory dyslexia. Her teacher has begun to suspect that she does not perceive word elements accurately. Because she is a resourceful person, the teacher has devised a simple listening test to estimate Mary's perceptual accuracy. Below is a sample of the child's performance.

Mary, listen carefully as I say each set of words. Tell me *Alike* if the two words are exactly the same. Tell me *Different* if the words are not exactly the same.

Pronounced by Teacher	*Mary's Responses*
"bed – dead"	Different
"dime – time"	Alike
"back – pack"	Alike
"look – look"	Alike

"tam – dam"	Alike
"pane – bane"	Alike
"dill – bill"	Different
"say – say"	Alike
"fat – vat"	Alike
"no – no"	Alike
"hot – what"	Alike
"vetch – fetch"	Alike
"mile – Nile"	Different
"where – hare"	Alike
"got – got"	Alike

A frustrating tendency is sometimes encountered in an activity of this nature. Many dyslexics do not follow instructions well enough to respond with the stereotyped phrases expected by the teacher. Instead of saying "Alike" or "Different," Mary might say "Yes" or "No," or "Same" and "Not the Same." Such behavior should not be regarded as incorrect. The point is to find out whether the child perceives sounds accurately, not whether he parrots back stereotyped answer codes. Much of the misery in the classroom between dyslexics and teachers results from the adult's failure to interpret the child's confused signals correctly.

This kind of informal diagnosis reveals some significant deficiences in Mary's auditory perception. The teacher now has definite guidelines for corrective teaching. This brief activity has revealed the child's confusion with four sets of similar sound elements: /d/ and /t/; /b/ and /p/; /f/ and /v/; /h/ and /hw/. The teacher will be alert for other areas of faulty perception as she guides Mary's reading and spelling growth. Teachers, however, must be cautious in placing faith in the results of tests like this. Many auditory dyslexics can make perfect scores on such oral-aural screening instruments. A score on an auditory discrimination test neither establishes nor eliminates a dyslexic condition until other symptoms are also identified (see checklist at end of chapter).

Confusion with Spelling

Auditory dyslexia is usually the primary cause for habitually poor spelling. Because the student does not distinguish discrete sounds accurately, he has no dependable way to remember how to spell. Traditional spelling instruction has been seriously detrimental to auditory dyslexics. When an arbitrary list of unrelated word forms is assigned on Monday, to be memorized however the child can for Friday's dictation test, the dyslexic student is faced with a frustrating predicament. Intelligent dyslexics frequently devise their own mnemonic systems for remembering spelling patterns. ("When" is h–e–n with *w* in front. "Mother" is t–h–e with *mo* in front and *r* at the end.) Today's curriculum involving the child with thousands of words at an ever accelerating pace soon produces impossible demands. Few individuals are clever enough to achieve literacy through mnemonic devices alone.

One of the surest symptoms of auditory dyslexia is chronic erasing, crossing out, or marking over (overprinting) to correct written mistakes. A careful observer soon discerns why dyslexics stagger through writing activities so nervously. A dyslexic writer "thinks out loud" as he works, mumbling to himself, studying his encoded thoughts, recognizing or imagining spelling errors, erasing and then writing another combination of letter symbols, never sure he has spelled correctly. Handwriting is an intensely personal manifestation of any writer's self. This is especially so for the insecure student who has never been able to please his teachers. Every word committed to paper exposes the dyslexic to probable failure. He faces this chronic risk nervously; therefore, he erases again and again, desperately trying to "luck out" with the correct combinations of letters, hoping to please his critics but not really expecting to succeed. Many dyslexic students attempt to hide their work as they write, a further indication of their dread of failure.

Certain patterns of error characterize the spelling efforts of auditory dyslexics. Classroom teachers do not need to purchase special tests to diagnose this disability. Four basic patterns of error will be apparent, regardless of the source of the dictation.

Transposed Consonant Elements. Dyslexics habitually change consonant patterns. "Barn" becomes *bran,* "play" becomes *paly,* and "girl" becomes *gril,* in many cases. The student seldom recognizes these transpositions because of his basic difficulty in associating sound units with their written symbols.

Phonetic Spellings. It is almost impossible for auditory dyslexics to apply phonic generalizations to spelling. When attempting to translate what they hear into written form, disabled students usually grope for literal translations. Teachers can detect this tendency if the student's garbled writing is read phonetically. In his attempts to encode familiar words, the dyslexic often writes "reefews" for *refuse,* or "gard" for *guard.* The old cliché that a child cannot spell cat is sometimes true. Many dyslexics write "kat" for *cat* and "cind" for *kind.*

Sound Units Omitted. The most significant indicator of auditory dyslexia in spelling is the habit of leaving out sound units within multisyllable words. This problem is sometimes called telescoping (see
Glossary). The following examples illustrate this tendency.

Dictated by Teacher	Student's Written Response
remember	rember
extravagance	exstragunce
tuberculosis	toberkulous
candidacy	candiacy
indefinitely	endefinely

Sound Units Added. A further characteristic of auditory dyslexia is
the tendency to add unnecessary sound units when encoding words. This
is also called perseveration (see Glossary). This tendency is illustrated
by this specimen.

Dictated by Teacher	Student's Written Response
duck	dukey
pretty	patting
party	paturing
doll	dalken
blizzard	blizzered
successful	sucessiful
immediate	immediant
intimate	intament
legitimate	lagetiment
zephyr	zesphir

Following is an effective fifteen-word dictation test, devised by Dr.
Ernest Jones.[1] This simple diagnostic instrument allows a teacher or
clinician to detect dyslexic symptoms quickly and accurately, as illustrated
by the following specimens.

A more complete diagnostic picture for older students can be obtained from word lists utilizing multisyllable words. A widely used
standardized spelling test is from the Metropolitan Achievement Tests.

---

[1] This test is used by permission of Dr. Ernest Jones. The test was used as a
screening device at Central State University for several years. It is not copyrighted.

dig	deg	dig	dit
for	for	for	for
pig	pig	pig	pig
barn	brne	brnu	bar
say	sae	Say	sand
pretty	pette	prite	patting
kind	cide	cind	kin
brown	bown	brond	brown
party	prtte	prtey	patwing
on	on	on	no
duck	Dirk	dukey	duck
bear	Bare	beru	bru
doll	Dall	dill	dalken
ate	ate	ate	eat
goes	gose	gos	gose

Metropolitan Achievement Tests:
Spelling List: Form S

Metropolitan Achievement Tests:
Spelling List: Form R

raise	*rase*
toward	*tword*
remember	*rember*
doubtful	*doughtful*
customer	*coustamer*
blizzard	*blizzred*
successful	*successful*
journal	*jurnel*
registration	*redustration*
edition	*edishon*
sincerely	*senseorly*
sensible	*senoable*
annual	*anuel*
faculty	*factualy*
alcohol	*achoal*
ambitious	*ambeshous*

source	*sorce*
response	*resporce*
session	*secesion*
extension	*efstention*
immediate	*immdeant*
affectionately	*affectionitly*
intimate	*intament*
achievement	*achivement*
efficient	*effecent*
extravagance	*extravagance*
tuberculosis	*toberkulous*
candidacy	*candeacy*
adieu	*adue*
legitimate	*logetiment*
indefinitely	*endefinely*
zephyr	*zesphir*

Above are samples of spelling efforts by high school students, illustrating the fact that auditory dyslexia is not a problem which children simply outgrow.[2]

---

[2] These specimens are from the 1946 copyright edition of the Metropolitan Achievement Tests, used by permission of the publisher. This edition has been superceded by a more recent edition, published by Harcourt Brace Jovanovich, Inc.

A simple spelling test is presented in Appendix B. This subtest of the JWST (Jordan Written Screening Test) is a carefully arranged group of words which are commonly misspelled by dyslexics. In a few minutes of group time the teacher can identify dyslexics without causing embarrassment. The following specimen illustrates how this dictation test reveals confusion with symbols as well as specific dyslexic tendencies to reverse, rotate, and transpose symbols.

1. dig	*dig*	14. pig	*pig*	27. big	*big*
2. ate	*eat*	15. rode	*rode*	28. goes	*goos*
3. play	*play*	16. please	*plei's*	29. toes	*tove*
4. duck	*duck*	17. buck	*buck*	30. track	*track*
5. party	*pardy*	18. pretty	*play*	31. try	*try*
6. brown	*drown*	19. born	*bon*	32. for	*foe*
7. barn	*bone*	20. brand	*brand*	33. from	*from*
8. girl	*gral*	21. bird	*bred*	34. stop	*stop*
9. saw	*sow*	22. was	*woe*	35. post	*post*
10. kind	*croned*	23. king	*king*	36. slat	*slit*
11. city	*ciy*	24. cent	*sent*	37. salt	*slat*
12. this	*this*	25. think	*thienk*	38. how	*how*
13. on	*an*	26. no	*no*	39. who	*who*

Auditory dyslexia is a major handicap when disabled students attempt to write essay answers or produce original stories or themes. Dyslexic spelling is frequently associated with dysgraphia (see Chapter 4). It is not difficult to discover the symptoms of auditory dyslexia in a student's written work, if classroom teachers analyze handwritten papers carefully.

Following is an example of dyslexic writing by a bright girl in Grade Four. Her autobiography was brushed aside as the work of a retarded child until her teacher discovered that the girl was dyslexic, not retarded. This specimen illustrates a combination of auditory dyslexia (faulty sound-symbol association) and dysgraphia (inability to write legibly).

Following the handwriting is a translation to illustrate the auditory dyslexic spelling flaws more clearly.

I was born in califarna (California) S (I) in (am) ten years old my brothers are six and four my dog is three years old my parents are 34 and 33 years old I like my parents wery (very) much my dad is in watnam (Vietnam) he will come home in about 3 months we have a geny (Guinea) pig it is three years old and i got a turdle (turtle) it is aloud (about) a week old S (I) like my turdle he dosnt (doesn't) lite (bite) some times the geny pig lites (bites) but mot (not) very much. my dog doesn't bite ever unless its a rolber (robber). one tine (time) vhen (when) i was in south

america a ruller (robber) tried to get in the door my dog barked
and scared the rillers (robbers) away and lm (I'm) glad to be in
the united states. my brothers names are robert and Mike may
(my) dogs (dog's) name is Oueen (Queen) my gene pig is sweat
peat (Sweet Pete) and i dont now (know) what to call the turdle.

No one knows how many intelligent, creative students have been written
off as academic failures because adults have not known how to identify
perceptual impairment. Below is the work of an intelligent teen-ager
who had been assigned to a class for mentally retarded children. When
an alert teacher studied his written work, she discovered that auditory
dyslexia and dysgraphia were his handicaps, not mental retardation. With
corrective training he completed a four-year college program.

READING INTEREST INVENTORY

Name *J. D.*   Age *14*   Grade in School *9th*

1. What do you usually do after school? *I go home ands golf for*
   a little wile and watch T.V.
2. What do you usually do on weekends? *goes golfing or fishing or sides*

3. What do you usually do during the summer? *to go golf and camping*

4. Who is your favorite TV or movie actor/actress? *Jack Weab*
   John Uane, and many more
5. What is your favorite kind of movie? *Crame*

6. What do you like best about school? *athletics*

7. What do you like least about school? *Science*

8. What kinds of hobbies do you enjoy doing? *Coins colleting*

9. Where have you been on trips? *to Miosouri, Arkansas, Kanasa,*
   new Myuico, Airjoma, Nevea, and California
10. How often do you check books out of the library? *very sledem*

11. What kinds of books do you like best to read? *books about pernons*
    that were famous and I like to read stapts
12. What magazines come to your home? *Sports Lillestrad*

A poorly administered intelligence test labeled another boy with
an IQ of 72. He was assigned to a class for borderline mentally retarded
students in high school. When his dyslexic handicap was diagnosed,

Larry's mental ability was correctly measured as above average. The following excerpt is from a manuscript he sent to a publisher.

> *The next morning, Gorge was the first one up and came over and wock me up because he heard a baing nose out side shureenuff they where taben allthe good stuf out of the car and when they got through they pored gasalen allover the car and left the cans inthe car. When*

Larry sent five original story manuscripts to a major paperback publisher. To his astonishment an enterprising editor deciphered the poor handwriting (dysgraphia) and discovered the story lines Larry had created. The editor returned the manuscripts with a lengthy critique, advising the boy what to do to improve the stories. He encouraged Larry to keep sending in story ideas, pointing out that the publisher was interested in purchasing fresh story materials. With this unique incentive, Larry became interested in school achievement. It is a sobering thought that this bright young man had been labeled hopeless by teachers who had not recognized the potential behind his disability.

Confusion with Rhyming Elements

An easily detected characteristic of auditory dyslexia is difficulty with rhyme. As a standard practice in elementary reading instruction, most teachers dwell on rhyming word entities to reinforce pupil awareness of certain aspects of phonics. Children handicapped by auditory dyslexia have great difficulty comprehending likenesses and differences in word elements. Awkwardness in identifying or reproducing rhymes is a major symptom of this disability.

Educators probably make too great an issue of faulty rhyming ability. Aside from providing a convenient vehicle for phonics drills, rhyming skill is actually of little practical importance, so far as overall reading maturity is concerned. The ability to rhyme, however, does help many children master writing and spelling. It is unfortunate that children with poor rhyming skill are penalized.

Item 18 on the JWST (see Appendix B) provides a simple test which allows the classroom teacher to detect faulty rhyming quickly. It should be remembered that many children who do oral rhyming activities well cannot do so in written form. To be sure of the extent of the disability, the teacher must use both oral and written activities.

An example of this informal procedure is to ask the child to name all the words he can which rhyme with "car." A child with normal perception should respond quickly with such words as "jar, far, star, bar." If the child finds this awkward, needing considerable time to ponder through each word before saying it, he may be handicapped by auditory dyslexia. This will be particularly evident if he names nonsense words, such as "dar, sar, nar, har, zar." Dyslexics often name words that begin alike but do not rhyme, such as "car, care, core, cure." If the student is unable to match printed rhyming word forms, or if he is unable to write down familiar rhyming words by substituting beginning consonants, the teacher can be reasonably sure that an auditory dyslexic condition exists.

Need for Speaker to Repeat

An especially irritating factor for many teachers is the dyslexic's need for repetition. Perceptually impaired students are insecure, particularly within an academic context. Auditory dyslexics are especially ill at ease in school because of their inability to comprehend sound-symbol associations accurately. When writing from dictation (auditory-to-motor) or following a series of oral instructions, the dyslexic student simply cannot cope with a sustained flow of oral material. Because of his extremely slow rate in transcribing speech into written form, the auditory dyslexic loses the sequence of oral elements.

Since they are never sure that they have heard accurately, dyslexics continuously ask the speaker to repeat. This habit produces friction in many learning situations. As disabled students chronically fall behind their peers, they tend to become disruptive. Chronic discipline problems often stem from the subtle, invisible presence of perceptual impairment. It is not unusual for dyslexics to be ostracized by their peers who are annoyed by their "weird" behavior and disruptive habits. Struggling to hold their social position creates chronic friction, which results in habitual conflict with adult authority. What begins as a perceptual flaw often leads to social jeopardy and public embarrassment. Yet little of this poor behavior is deliberate on the part of dyslexics.

Subvocalizing during Silent Reading

A common stereotype of primary teachers is the crisp snapping of fingers, followed by "Shhhhhhhh!" For many years children have been taught that making vocal sounds during silent reading time is forbidden. Perhaps this practice does enhance learning for certain youngsters, although it is probably more beneficial to the teacher's frazzled nerves than to growth in reading skills. The truth is that dyslexic students *must* subvocalize, if they are to succeed in translating writing into meaningful thought. Because of the underlying problem in associating sounds with written symbols, dyslexic readers must use a variety of stimulus channels to verify their decoding impressions. A child with no impairment can learn to decode through visual stimulus alone (6). A perceptually impaired child cannot.

This frustrating need to reinforce visual cues with vocal response, along with the tactile impression of following words with a finger on the page, should not upset classroom teachers. As suggested in Chapter 6, it is not difficult to allow handicapped children to respond in their unorthodox ways if the teacher is aware of the problem. The important consideration is that dyslexic children must respond to reading in a variety of ways in order to check their impressions for accuracy. When the teacher snaps her fingers and hisses "Shhhhhhh!" she is cutting off an essential learning channel for auditory dyslexics. The result can only be increased frustration and failure.

This need to reinforce symbol translation with vocal and tactile response also appears when auditory dyslexics are engaged in written assignments. These students need to subvocalize during spelling tests, or while writing stories or essays. If dyslexics are allowed to cross-check their impressions of oral and written symbols, they can learn to correct many mistakes in reading and spelling.

Difficulty Blending Parts into Word Wholes

In Chapter 1 an example was given of Mary's attempt to read aloud from a science text. The heart of her decoding handicap is faulty blending, which leaves her unable to cope with one of the major skills of accurate word analysis. The entire auditory dyslexic syndrome seems to focus upon Mary's problems in "sounding out" words as she reads. For example, a familiar word like "bug" can become a major hurdle for the dyslexic reader. Laboriously Mary breaks the word apart: "buh–uh–guh." As this effort illustrates, she has never accurately identified the vocal production for the consonants b and g. When she feels somewhat confident that she has the separate elements in mind, Mary takes the plunge: "Blug." Again she has failed. "Yellow" comes out yelelow, and "bridge" turns into burge. Children like Mary quickly grow defensive and insecure when forced to expose themselves to such public failure.

Traditional instruction in phonics which emphasizes blending is usually beyond the comprehension of auditory dyslexics. It is possible for students like Mary to achieve success in simple word analysis after long-range drill and rote memorization of key word patterns. This technique, called overteaching, saturates the child with intensive, highly structured practice with regular word forms until an automatic response occurs. Children like Mary seldom come to a true understanding of blending and word analysis, although they can often achieve an independent level of reading.

Garbled Pronunciation

Closely associated with the inability to blend is an embarrassing problem of garbled pronunciation. Auditory dyslexics find themselves the object of much laughter and teasing because of scrambled articulation. Classroom teachers can identify this aspect of dyslexia by devising lists of words for the child to repeat. This faulty articulation is also referred to as *echolalia* (see Glossary).

Normal Pronunciation	Auditory Dyslexic Response
aluminum	alunimum
vinegar	vigenar
animals	aminals
olive	olly
baskets	baksets
streamline	steamline
spaghetti	pasghetti

Teachers and students can have fun with pronunciation games which reveal echolalia, the garbled speech in which strategic sound units are transposed within words. For example, the teacher might devise a "Tongue Twister Race," keeping a diagnostic record of garbled speech tendencies of certain children. The emphasis must be upon fun with no child feeling shame because of a twisted tongue.

Below are some good word combinations for this informal diagnosis:

"apples in cinnamon"   "aluminum animals"
"alum in vinegar"   "Mama's spaghetti"
"baskets of olives"   "transcontinental train"
"she sells sea shells on the seashore"

Older students enjoy such twisters as these:

"political candidacy"
"musketry maneuvers"

"blueberry strudel"
"a crow flew over the river with a lump of raw liver"
"six long, slim, sleek, slick, slender saplings"

Confusion with Dictionary Symbols

As would be expected, the auditory dyslexia syndrome makes traditional dictionary usage quite difficult for handicapped students. Problems in encoding and decoding make reading and writing hazardous activities. To expect dyslexics to interpret phonetic respellings, accent markings, and pronunciation code systems is beyond their reach, as a rule. Intelligent, highly motivated students with perceptual limitations do manage to cope with the various codes found in reference materials. Most dyslexic children, however, cannot comprehend the variety of symbol systems they encounter in current dictionaries. This problem is further complicated by the current use of ambiguous schwa symbols showing vowel sounds in unaccented syllables. Dyslexic students can benefit from studies in word origins, multiple meanings, and syllable division, but to arrive at correct word pronunciations from dictionary keys is frequently impossible.

Checklist of Auditory Dyslexia Symptoms

There is danger in attaching labels to student behavior, particularly labels which denote disability or impaired ability to learn. Some students appear dyslexic who actually suffer hearing loss, or who have never been taught good study habits. A speech impediment can produce poor articulation which resembles auditory dyslexia. In spite of these dangers, the following checklist can help classroom teachers identify clusters of behavior which are associated with auditory dyslexia. It is important that teachers withhold judgment until a definite syndrome of symptoms has been identified.

_____Confusion with Phonics

_____Cannot distinguish differences in vowel sounds

_____does not perceive long vowel sounds

_____does not perceive short vowel sounds

_____does not perceive schwa vowel sounds

_____does not comprehend variant vowel sounds

_____Cannot distinguish differences in consonant sounds

_____does not perceive differences between similar consonant sounds:

_____/b/ /d/   _____/b/ /p/
_____/d/ /t/   _____/g/ /k/
_____/m/ /n/   _____/f/ /v/
_____/s/ /z/   _____/th/ /f/

_____does not identify elements within consonant clusters

_____Cannot interpret diacritical markings

_____Cannot interpret phonetic respellings

_____Confusion with Words

_____Cannot tell when words are alike or different

_____Cannot detect or reproduce rhyming words

_____Gives garbled pronunciation (echolalia)

_____Confusion with Spelling

_____Writes very slowly

_____Depends upon mnemonic devices to recall spellings

_____Is not able to apply phonic generalizations when spelling

_____Tends to spell phonetically

_____Breaks consonant clusters when spelling (transposes l and r)

_____Confuses sound values of consonant letters:

_____c for k   _____f for v
_____m for n   _____d for t
_____s for z   _____f for th

_____Does not perceive sounds of /m/, /n/, /l/, /w/, or /r/

_____Leaves out sound units when writing words (telescopes)

_____Adds sound units when writing words (perseverates)

_____Does not perceive accent in words

_____Does not perceive vowel sounds within words

_____Does not perceive syllables within words

_____Does not remember variant or unusual spellings

_____Is not able to retain memory stock of basic spelling words

_____Asks speaker to repeat

_____Erases, marks over, crosses out

_____Attempts to hide work while writing

_____Reinforcement While Writing or Reading

_____Whispers (subvocalizes) while reading silently

_____Whispers (subvocalizes) while writing

References for Further Reading

1. Baker, G.A.P. "Behavior Problem or Auditory Interfererences (sic)?" *Academic Therapy Quarterly* 6 (Summer 1971): 385-389.

2. Doehring, D. G., and Rabinovitch, M. S. "Auditory Abilities of Children with Learning Problems." *Journal of Learning Disabilities* 2 (September 1969): 467-475.

3. Eakin, Suzanne, and Douglas, V. I. "Automatization and Oral Reading Problems in Children." *Journal of Learning Disabilities* 4 (January 1971): 26-33.

4. Gibson, Eleanor J., and Levin, Harry. *The Psychology of Reading.* pp. 340-351. Cambridge, Massachusetts: The M.I.T. Press, 1975.

5. Golden, N. E., and Steiner, S. R. "Auditory and Visual Functions in Good and Poor Readers." *Journal of Learning Disabilities* 2 (September 1969): 476-481.

6. Holloway, G. F. "Auditory-Visual Integration in Language-Delayed Children." *Journal of Learning Disabilities* 4 (April 1971): 204-208.

7. Johnson, Doris J., and Myklebust, Helmer R. *Learning Disabilities: Educational Principles and Practices,* New York: Grune & Stratton, 1967.

8. Kinsbourne, Marcel, and Warrington, E. K. "Disorders of Spelling." *The Disabled Reader: Education of the Dyslexic Child.* Edited by John Money, pp. 73-81. Baltimore: The Johns Hopkins Press, 1966.

9. Wagenberg, Renee, and Blau, Harold. "Hyperlexia: The Problem of the Wordy Child." *Academic Therapy Quarterly* 6 (Summer 1971): 411-412.

10. Weiner, P. S. "The Cognitive Functioning of Language Deficient Children." *Cognitive Studies: Deficits in Cognition.* Edited by Jerome Hellmuth. Vol. 2, pp. 338-350. New York: Brunner/Mazel Publishers, 1971.

chapter 4

Dysgraphia in the Classroom

HANDWRITING IS A SENSITIVE PERSONAL MATTER. UNDER CERTAIN conditions graphologists may introduce handwriting analysis as court evidence, testifying that one's script is a unique signature of the writer's personality. Partly because of its personal nature, penmanship practice has been one of the least popular school activities, particularly among boys. In the present curriculum a trend is developing to remove pressure from primary pupils to perfect their handwriting; the students are no longer expected to fill pages with push-pulls and smoke screens, remembered well by older persons. Gradually teachers seem to be accepting uniqueness in student penmanship, so long as the writing is legible.

Ironically, old-fashioned penmanship drills may have remediated a form of dyslexia which is a growing educational problem in modern classrooms. Since the advent of manuscript printing in primary grades, many intelligent youngsters have not learned to write acceptably. Fifty years ago stereotyped penmanship drills saturated children with perceptual awareness of letter formation. Today increasing thousands of students are writing failures.

The inability to cope with handwriting is called dysgraphia. This term refers to difficulty in producing legible handwriting. Dysgraphia involves faulty control of the muscle systems used to encode letters and word forms accurately. The dysgraphic student usually has a clear mental image of what he intends to encode, but he finds himself "forgetting" how to write specific symbols. Certain letters are made with backward or upside-down motions. Handwriting is generally so awkward and unsatisfactory that dysgraphic students avoid situations where they have to practice penmanship whenever possible.

Many dysgraphic persons do learn to read acceptably. Dysgraphia, however, is generally associated with both visual and auditory dyslexia.

Teachers and clinicians seldom see one form of dyslexia which is not complicated to some degree by other symptoms of impairment. When seriously dysgraphic children are permitted to use alternate means of encoding, such as typewriters or dictation machines, handwriting disability can be largely ignored as an educational problem. So long as educators insist that all children master legible cursive style, dysgraphia will continue to be a frustrating educational handicap.

Dysgraphia Syndrome

It is important that teachers distinguish between careless handwriting habits and perceptual impairment. Boys often reject the restrictions of attractive writing style. Since teachers tend to judge student competence by the neatness of written work, dysgraphic students are at a serious disadvantage. There are definite characteristics which differentiate dysgraphia from carelessness. This problem is not difficult to diagnose in the classroom, in view of the wide variety of handwriting specimens available from each student's quota of written work handed in for evaluation.

Difficulty Learning Alphabet Forms

The primary characteristic of dysgraphia is the student's difficulty in remembering how to form certain letters. The classroom teacher might not identify this flaw unless she watches the child write. Cursive writing style is intended to flow from left to right. Dysgraphia involves the tendency to work backwards, from right to left. So long as primary pupils print isolated letter forms in manuscript style, this backward tendency presents a rather minor problem because the letters are not connected in series. Dysgraphia becomes a crippling factor as children are expected to develop skill in left-to-right cursive writing style, usually taught in Grade Three.

Few adults seem aware of the staggering perceptual burden modern education has placed upon beginner pupils, so far as the written symbol system of our language is concerned. Adults who have attained literacy and handwriting fluency tend to regard primary education as the mastery of twenty-six alphabet letter forms. Unfortunately this is a false conception of primary instruction. Since the early 1930s American educators have taught manuscript print in Grade One. Yet the alphabetic sequence (A through Z) is not taught, as a rule. Instead of learning twenty-six letter forms, primary pupils are expected to master two sets of alphabet symbols, including capital and lowercase forms, for a total of at least 104 alphabet symbols. Since many manuscript capital letters are distinctly different from lowercase letters, the beginner pupil must learn fifty-two letter forms in manuscript style, not twenty-six. Later, when the transition is made to cursive style, fifty-two new letter forms must be learned, bringing the total to 104.

Manuscript print is usually continued throughout Grade Two. All of this time young readers are exposed to a wide variety of type styles in their reading materials. The Library of Congress lists more than 100 different typefaces commonly found in leisure reading materials in America. Near the end of Grade Two, or by the middle of Grade Three, children are told in effect that manuscript style will no longer be satisfactory. Now they must forget all that they have learned and learn a new style of letter and word formation. The fifty-two isolated, unconnected letter forms mastered through hours and days of drill are now gradually discarded while a new handwriting style, called cursive, is introduced. As with manuscript print, cursive style utilizes not just the twenty-six letters but rather fifty-two new forms, although there is similarity between several capital and lowercase symbols. By the beginning of Grade Four the primary pupil is expected to have learned to encode from memory 104 alphabet forms, which includes the unlearning of two years' work learning the concepts of manuscript letter formation.

Along with learning to cope with fifty-two manuscript symbols, primary pupils are simultaneously confronted by more than thirty printer's cues (see Glossary) commonly used in basal readers, library books, textbooks, and other sources of reading in elementary classrooms. Youngsters are expected to distinguish several marks of punctuation, color cues, boldface type, italics, indentation, chapter and story headings, unique page format, and myriad other symbols included in the repertoire of beginning reading skills. These symbol systems take on meaning only when the youngster has successfully mastered their relationships with his speaking and listening language. Few adults would willingly attempt such a staggering burden of symbol mastery within a three-year span. The wonder is not that many children fail; the wonder is that so many succeed.

To begin a child's quest for literacy with manuscript printing is heavily defended by most educators as a feasible educational practice. This author, however, has yet to see convincing evidence that such a temporary, transitional symbol system is worth two years of investment of teacher and pupil time. The fact that most students achieve literacy may vindicate the use of manuscript writing in beginning instruction. The fact remains that this educational practice is a serious barrier for handicapped children who are more confused than edified by 104 alphabet symbols within a three-year span.

Dysgraphia becomes a crippling factor as it brings the student into conflict with tradition, particularly the left-to-right pattern of American literacy. The more difficult cursive letter forms for dysgraphic children are those involving closed, circular elements (such as $d, b, p, g, f, g, a, e, o$). Equally difficult are letters requiring a change in direction of hand movement (such as c, h, f, t, z). Dysgraphics frequently have difficulty remembering where to stop a sweeping or circular movement, how to swing back, and how to connect the lines of movement within complicated letter formations ($A, B, D, F, H, K, J, M, n, U, W, X$). The dysgraphic writer has great difficulty remembering where and how to stop circular motions in order to swing accurately into the next letter when spelling out words. The difficulties are dramatically minimized when children are drilled in connected cursive style instead of in isolated manuscript forms.

Classroom teachers must develop two skills of observation if they are to detect dysgraphia quickly. The teacher must actually observe the child at work. Dysgraphics often mask their difficulties so that the handicap may not be apparent on sample papers the teacher collects for evaluation. It is also essential for the teacher to learn to re-create the child's writing style by tracing over the student's handwriting slowly, observing the flaws in directionality and discovering where the writing breaks down for the child.

Presented are two specimens of writing by an intelligent girl in Grade Four. The first specimen is Glenda's attempt to write the alphabet from memory. This illustrates her confusion in transferring from manuscript to cursive style, as indicated by the mixture of the two styles in her writing. Dysgraphia is noted by her difficulty in forming the loops on d, b, and p. She also confuses d and b because of her initial experiences with these letter forms in isolated, unconnected manuscript style. Capital Z causes Glenda considerable confusion, as indicated by her erasures and awkward overprinting. By tracing over this child's writing attempt, the reader can feel the dyslexic confusion Glenda experiences.

Dysgraphia can become evident as the classroom teacher reviews written exercises done by her pupils. Below is a spelling exercise which Glenda wrote from dictation. Any specimen of written work can be used to screen for dysgraphia. The reader should trace slowly over Glenda's writing, saying the words over and over while tracing, just as Glenda mumbled the words as she wrote. Small arrows beside the letters indicate the backward motions this dysgraphic student uses in writing. This chronic reversal pattern illustrates why Glenda is an extremely slow, insecure writer.

A careful observer will note the many broken letters in Glenda's writing. Her cursive word forms are actually a series of pieces she has

big	duck
for	bear
pig	doll
barn	ate
say	goes
pretty	play
kind	
brown	
party	
on	

strung together in imitation of word models she has seen. In words like "pig" that begin with p, she starts at the bottom, marking upward, and ending in a backward loop to form the top. Since this causes her to finish inside the word, she is forced to break the continuity by arbitrarily starting the next letter somewhere near the bottom loop on p. Initial f is also patched together because she does not recall how and when to change the direction of her hand movements.

This lack of continuity causes Glenda to circle again and again when writing d, b, a, o, and e, as illustrated in the words barn, brown, party, duck, bear, doll, ate, goes, and play. The reader can easily imagine the near panic this child experiences during pressured writing activities in school.

A more serious form of dysgraphia is illustrated below in the writing of a highly intelligent boy in Grade Three. This pupil's work is handicapped by a combination of visual dyslexia and dysgraphia, as revealed by the reversed letters and word elements. These dyslexic tendencies were almost entirely corrected during a fourteen-week cycle of intensive training which supplemented his regular classroom activities. The key to success was his mastery of cursive writing. The child practiced an hour each day until he had mastered the cursive lowercase alphabet in connected sequence. As alphabetical order and sequence became automatic, the dysgraphic problems shown below began to disappear. By the end of Grade Three this child was meeting grade-level expectations in writing and spelling from dictation.

dig

for

pig

barn

say

pretty

kind

brown

party

on

duck

bear

doll

ate

goes

Mirror Writing

An interesting form of dysgraphia is commonly called "mirror writing" (see Glossary). True mirror writing can actually be read when held up to a mirror. A complete mirror image is rarely encountered by classroom teachers, but varying degrees of this tendency are commonly found in dysgraphic work. As a rule, only certain words or portions of words will be written backwards. The counterpart of mirror writing is mirror reading, in which whole words are read from right to left ("was" for saw, "tub" for but, "no" for on).

Below is an example of mirror writing done by Vanessa, a bright child in Grade Two. At first Vanessa's teacher was perplexed by this handwriting. Not only was this the young lady's first year of teaching, but also none of her professional education courses had mentioned mirror writing or any other form of dyslexia. Vanessa did not exhibit mirror tendencies in reading. Because she had partially adjusted to the left-to-

Dictated by Teacher

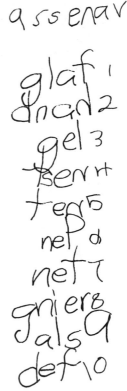

1. flag

2. hand

3. leg

4. nest

5. nut

6. pen

7. ten

8. ring

9. sled

10. fed

right sequence, she was able to overcome her tendency to mirror write rather quickly when the teacher understood the nature of the handicap.

Sentence Structure as a Guide

A significant clue to a dysgraphic student's language potential is sentence structure, or syntax, which is largely camouflaged by poorly executed handwriting. Two examples of frustrated creativity are presented below. The passages have been translated to illustrate the language maturity of each child. In each case an interested teacher took time to decipher the messy, crudely executed handwriting which at first glance seemed not worth wading through. When the perceptual impairment had been recognized, these children were no longer regarded as "lazy" and "care-

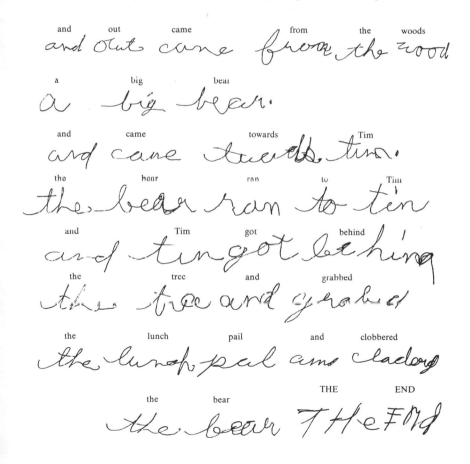

less." They made rapid improvement through the supplemental hand-writing guidance their teachers provided in the classroom.

The first specimen (p. 00) is Donna's response to an unfinished story in *From Faraway Places,* published by Harper and Row. After reading a brief story about children picking blueberries and being startled by "a loud, astonishing noise" from the woods, Donna was asked to imagine what happened next and then write an ending in her own words.

Andrew's Christmas story (below) represents a near tragedy in misdiagnosis according to surface evaluation of standardized scores. The WISC (Wechsler Intelligence Scale for Children) yielded these scores: Verbal IQ 103; Performance IQ 110; Full Scale IQ 107. He achieved Motor Age Equivalent 8.0 on the Bender Gestalt Test, six months above his chronological age. The Human Figure Drawing Completion Test yielded a score of 101 at the 53d percentile level. His handwriting, however, was virtually illegible in daily classroom work. The psychomotrist concluded that a severe emotional disturbance must exist. After all, it was reasoned, the motor indicators on the clinical tests "ruled out any sort of impairment in coordination."

The   first   Christmas

The First Christmas

Jesus   was   born   on   Christmas

Jesus was bain ane christmas

He   was   born   in   Bethlehem

Hit. he was ban in bilahmr

He   was   a   baby

He Was a baby

His   mother   was   named   Mary.

Hismtr was nal'y wbcs mre.

Jesus   preached   to   people.   He   was   crucified.

gh esas PLt to PePPji he wasc as a Fid.

This rigid reliance upon test scores was challenged by Andrew's classroom teacher who had noted a sophisticated language structure in the child's work. A reading diagnostician identified the problem as dysgraphia, which does not always show up on clinical tests for motor development. Older students helped the classroom teacher guide Andrew through daily supplemental training in handwriting skills. Within six weeks his dysgraphic symptoms had begun to disappear. This incident illustrates the danger involved when professionals look more at scores than at actual classroom performance of children.

The major flaw in Andrew's manuscript print is the broken letter pattern. Lowercase a, h, and m are usually fragmented, with the strokes scattered apart. This gives his writing the appearance of "bird scratches." Several letters are rotated toward the left, adding to the disoriented appearance of his work. These faults were remedied through practice in writing cursive style with letters connected in sequence.

Directionality

A crippling aspect of dyslexia is the inability to perceive parts of a whole in relation to the axis, or central position, of the whole. For example, students are expected to read horizontally from left to right. In writing, the hand is supposed to progress horizontally from left to right with the page tilted slightly toward the left. If a page is divided into columns, the student is expected to progress downward until his eyes or hand reach the bottom line, and then move directly upward and to the right for the next column. Since our entire culture is predicated upon the left-to-right, top-to-bottom orientation, anyone who perceives reading or writing differently is "wrong."

Left-handed writers frequently develop a legible writing style, although they appear to write upside down or backward. This unorthodox compensation of "lefties" has frustrated many penmanship teachers who feel that correct pen-to-shoulder alignment is a sacred ingredient for sound scholarship. But left-handed students have persisted in their unique writing styles, orthodox protests notwithstanding.

A subtle but common problem associated with dysgraphia is a confusion with horizontal and vertical directionality. Occasionally totally inverted perception is seen by clinicians. Such individuals read exactly upside down, perceiving symbols at 180 degrees rotation from "normal." Because these students are usually capable readers, their upside-down orientation is often not discovered in the classroom. This kind of skewed perception becomes a problem as children begin to adapt to typical perceptual style. Teachers frequently see certain students turning the page halfway around. Such behavior often indicates that the child perceives at ninety degrees rotation. For these readers the print becomes legible only when the rows of words are vertical, or ninety degrees from horizontal. This disorientation usually disappears as children are indoctrinated as to "correct orientation" concepts. The tendency seems to bother teachers more than it does the affected children.

Directional confusion does create a problem in handwriting, however. This form of dysgraphia is frequently camouflaged by extremely poor letter formation or by the generally messy appearance of the student's papers. As the dysgraphic student attempts to write, particularly with no visual model to follow, directional confusion creates erratic production, with much erasing and writing over, with blank spaces left if the student cannot cope with the task at all. In writing on unlined paper, the lines usually slant or wobble up and down from the horizontal axis, as illustrated in Donna's story ending about the bear. When moving from the bottom of one column to the top of the next, the writer sometimes exhibits a mirror perception of the vertical axis, writing on the left-hand side of the midline instead of on the right.

An example of this directional confusion is given below. Todd was a bright boy in Grade Two. His mental ability, as measured by the WISC, was Full Scale IQ 112, with thirty points discrepancy between Verbal and Performance IQ levels. This kind of discrepancy is frequently found in dysgraphic students. The following specimens are taken from his performance on the Slingerland Screening Tests for Identifying Children with Specific Language Disability: Form A (Revised Edition) for Grade I and Beginning Grade II.[1] The examples are from dictation tests which allowed no visual models for Todd to see or copy. He was working strictly from memory of letter forms and directionality (see pages 61 and 62).

Copying Simple Shapes

An earmark of dysgraphia is the inability to copy simple geometric shapes without distortion. This is often referred to as conservation of form. Teachers assume that children can hold mental images of what they see while those images are translated into fine muscle patterns for drawing or writing. Dysgraphia is the inability to do this complex perceptual task. Classroom teachers with limited budgets can use any activity with children involving copying circles, squares, diamonds, triangles, or rec-

---

[1] Educator's Publishing Service, Cambridge, Massachusetts 01238.

1. S r h

2. f d y

3. G DC

4. Pe vv h m is.

5. H bed Y m Ball

6. T h p

7. 1 2 10

8. C 0 l 6   "three twenty-six"

9. C me   "see me"

10. s p6   "to go"

11.   "he is"

12.   "my ball"

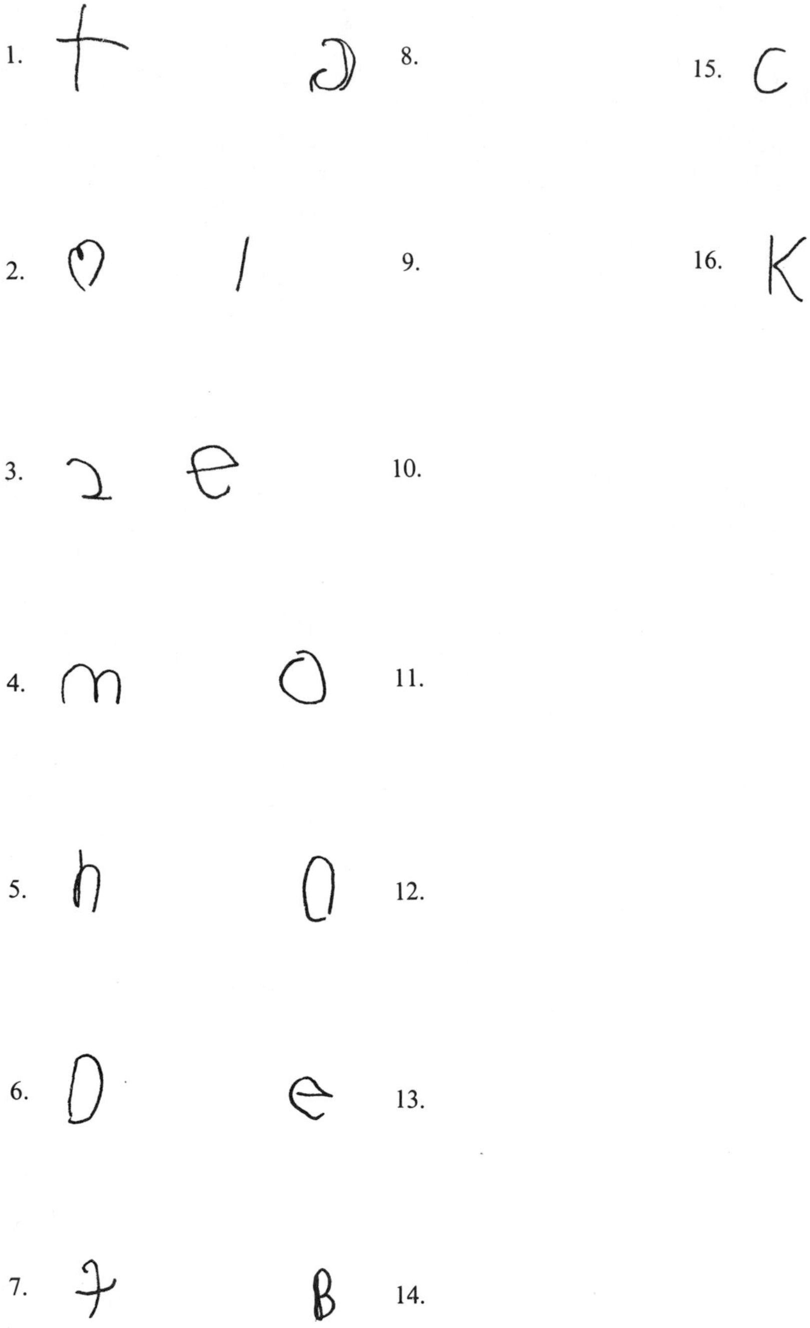

1. ✝   ə 8.   15. C

2. ♡   / 9.   16. K

3. ⊃   e 10.

4. m   O 11.

5. h   () 12.

6. D   e 13.

7. �   B 14.

tangles. It is important to allow for immaturity in younger children in primary grades. Dysgraphia is indicated only when other symptoms are also present in the child's handwriting and orientation tendencies.

Item 7 of the JWST (Jordan Written Screening Test) illustrates this dysgraphic tendency (see Appendix B). The following examples demonstrate how this simple activity reveals dysgraphic tendencies. This work was done by a student in Grade Six, Age 12–9, with mental ability within the average range.

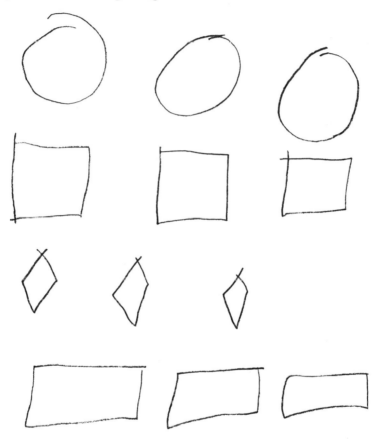

A frequently observed flaw in copying shapes is the tendency to draw "ears" at the corners of simple figures. Classroom teachers can observe this tendency in arithmetic exercises and art activities which involve students in sketching or copying shapes and figures. The following specimens of "ears" were observed while students were being given

the Stanford-Binet Intelligence Scale. Rather than indicating low intelligence, these failures represent perceptual impairment which was
eventually diagnosed as dysgraphia. Each student was asked to draw
a figure just like the one on the booklet. A model of a large diamond
was printed on the booklet for visual cues.

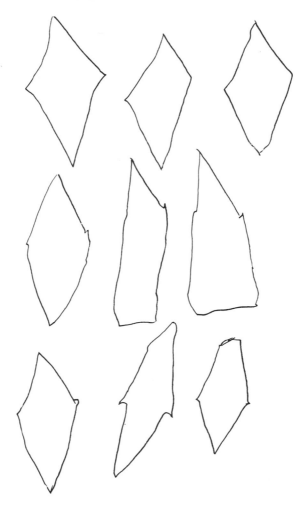

The Stanford-Binet Intelligence Scale contains another performance
item which is an especially accurate indicator of dysgraphic tendencies.
At the IX year, 3 month level, the student is presented with a card
which has two sketches. After studying the sketches for several seconds,
he is supposed to draw them from memory. Tendencies toward rotation

from the horizontal plane, as well as failure to observe minimal cues, are illustrated by the kinds of drawings shown below. When other dysgraphic characteristics are seen in the student's handwriting, this subtest of the Stanford-Binet is helpful in diagnosing dyslexia. In these examples, each child reversed the order (sequence) of the sketches, drawing the last one first.

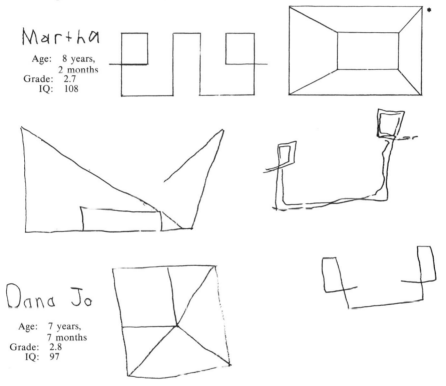

Martha
Age: 8 years, 2 months
Grade: 2.7
IQ: 108

Dana Jo
Age: 7 years, 7 months
Grade: 2.8
IQ: 97

* Reproduced by permission of the publisher, Houghton Mifflin Company.

Telescoping

When dysgraphic students are laboring to encode longer words, they commonly leave out portions of the letters or syllables without being aware of this error. The effort of putting down word units on paper is a laborious process for dysgraphics. After writing for a brief time, they tend to lose track of how much of a word form has been encoded. This habit is called telescoping (see Glossary), as illustrated in the spelling errors on page 38. Students who tend to telescope are usually handicapped by auditory dyslexia as well as dysgraphia.

Perseveration

The opposite of telescoping is perseveration (see Glossary). This problem involves the inability to turn loose of a pattern once the student has begun to produce a particular sequence. Perseveration is sometimes observed in oral reading or conversation when the speaker tends to repeat vocal patterns unnecessarily.

Occasionally perseveration occurs during rhyming drills, as when a child responds to "cat" by saying: "vat, dat, lat, nat, wat. . . ." This is not an effort to be amusing, in most cases. True perseveration is an involuntary reaction. The child is momentarily unable to stop his repeating reflex.

Dysgraphic children are often unable to halt the reproduction of certain letter or syllable patterns without completely stopping their work. Perseveration also results when children habitually lift their pencils from the paper midway through writing a word. This break in continuity leaves them unable to recall where they stopped in the word pattern.

Checklist of Dysgraphia Characteristics

This checklist can help classroom teachers distinguish between immaturity or poor instruction and perceptual impairment. It is important that judgment be withheld until an unmistakable cluster of dysgraphic symptoms has been identified in a child's handwriting behavior.

_____Difficulty with Alphabet or Number Symbols

_____Does not remember how to write certain letters or numerals

_____Distorts shapes of certain letters or numerals

_____Overall writing effort is awkward, uneven

_____Has difficulty transferring from manuscript to cursive style

_____Continues to print manuscript style long after introduction to cursive style

_____Fragments certain letter or numeral forms

_____Writing resembles "bird scratching"; is virtually illegible

_____Has difficulty distinguishing between capital and lowercase letter forms

_____Mixes capital and lowercase forms

_____Confusion with Directionality

_____Writes certain letters, numerals, or words in mirror image

_____Tends to write on mirror side (left side) of vertical

midline when moving to next column
_____Marks from bottom to top when forming certain letters or numerals
_____Uses backwards (clockwise) motions when forming loops in certain letters or numerals
_____Erases or overprints habitually to change directions of certain letters or numerals
_____Writing tends to slant up, down, or to wobble up and down

_____Sentence Structure

_____Composes meaningful content in spite of poor handwriting
_____Transposes grammatical elements within sentences, but produces good overall meaning
_____Tends to use complete sentence forms instead of fragments

_____Difficulty Conserving Form in Copying Simple Shapes

_____Distorts simple shapes
_____Fails to close corners
_____Draws "ears" where lines meet or change direction
_____Has difficulty reproducing simple designs from memory
_____Work deteriorates toward end of writing exercise
_____Has difficulty staying on lines when tracing

_____Tendency to Telescope

_____Omits letters when writing words
_____Omits syllables or sound units when writing words
_____Runs letters and words together
_____Runs words together (usually when copying)

_____Tendency to Perseverate

_____Adds unnecessary letters or sound units to written words
_____Repeats the same letters or syllables in written words
_____Adds unnecessary sound units to spoken words
Repeats syllables or sound units in spoken words
_____Falls into parrotlike repetition of rhyming units during games or conversation

References for Further Reading

1. Ball, T. S., *et al.* "The Orienting Response as a Nonverbal Measure of Body Awareness." *Cognitive Studies: Deficits in Cognition.* Edited by Jerome Hellmuth, vol. 2, pp. 351-363. New York: Brunner/Mazel Publishers, 1971.

2. Benson, D. F. "Graphic Orientation Disorders of Left-Handed Children." *Journal of Learning Disabilities* 3 (March 1970): 126-127.

3. Di Leo, J. H. *Young Children and Their Drawings.* New York: Brunner/Mazel Publishers, 1970.

4. Hearns, R. S. "Dyslexia and Handwriting." *Journal of Learning Disabilities* 2 (January 1969): 37-42.

5. Johnson, D. J., and Mykelbust, H. R. *Learning Disabilities: Educational Principles and Practices.* New York: Grune and Stratton, 1967.

6. Kaufman, Maurice. "Figure-Ground in Visual Perception." *Reading Disability and Perception.* Newark, Delaware: International Reading Association, Proceedings of the 13th Annual Convention, vol. 13, part 3 (1969): 119-126.

7. Kelly, G. R. "Group Perceptual Screening at First Grade Level." *Journal of Learning Disabilities* 3 (December 1970): 640-644.

8. Kershner, J. R. "Conservation of Multiple Space Relations by Children: Effects of Perception and Representation." *Journal of Learning Disabilities* 4 (June/July 1971): 316-321.

9. Kinsbourne, Marcel, and Warrington, E. K. "Developmental Factors in Reading and Writing Backwardness." *The Disabled Reader: Education of the Dyslexic Child.* Edited by John Money, pp. 59-71. Baltimore: The Johns Hopkins Press, 1966.

10. Rice, J. A. "Confusion in Laterality: A Validity Study with Bright and Dull Children." *Journal of Learning Disabilities* 2 (July 1969): 368-373.

11. Serio, Martha, and Anderson, Annetta. "Remedial Procedures from the Classroom: From Theory to Practice." *Academic Therapy Quarterly* 6 (Spring 1971): 321-325.

chapter 5

Correcting Visual Dyslexia in the Classroom

TEACHERS ARE FREQUENTLY ADVISED THERE IS NOTHING THEY CAN DO for dyslexics in the classroom. Many professionals contend that remediation of perceptual impairment is a job for specially trained clinicians. It is true that complex cases of dyslexia require the attention of specialists who have unique materials and equipment not available in regular classes. Most dyslexic students, however, can respond to corrective measures that are feasible within a typical classroom setting. When teachers are able to follow certain basic guidelines and establish flexible daily routines, most dyslexics can learn to cope with their handicaps without attending specialized clinics.

This book cannot include all the techniques for correcting dyslexia in the classroom. Interested teachers must tailor corrective techniques to fit the specific needs of their students. Presented here are guidelines and principles for working with dyslexic children. The activities used to illustrate the principles should serve as models. As in any teaching situation, classroom teachers must improvise according to their particular circumstances.

Principal 1: Self-fulfilling Prophecy

Much attention has been drawn by educators to the power a teacher's attitudes exert over the success or failure of her students. A general principle can be stated: "Students tend to accomplish what the teacher expects them to accomplish." In other words, students tend to return the feelings and attitudes they sense in their leaders. If the teacher expects her youngsters to succeed, they generally will do so. Positive teachers who respect their students are usually respected in return. Negative teachers who regard dyslexics as failures with little hope for success find these pupils failing in school, as well as displaying negative, disrespectful attitudes toward adults. Many studies reveal that test scores and achievement are closely tied to a teacher's personal expectations. In effect, the teacher who prophesies student success tends to see her pupils achieving success. The teacher who predicts failure and doom is not disappointed; her students tend to fail, thus fulfilling the teacher's prophecy.

Certainly there is more to success and failure than the teacher's expectations. But the attitude of the teacher is a critical factor for dyslexics. Certain adults are not temperamentally suited for working with disabled youngsters. When this is the case, the school should make every effort to give both teachers and students a choice. If working with dyslexics is offensive or uncomfortable for an adult, it will be impossible for a warm, accepting classroom relationship to be established. Students with disabilities do not respond positively to uncomfortable or rigid adults. More harm than good comes from forced associations between teachers who dread disabled children and students who are apprehensive toward their teachers. It is essential that classroom teachers have positive expectations concerning the potential abilities of handicapped students. If not, the association will be characterized by frustration, rebellion, anxiety, and failure.

Principle 2: What Does the Student Need?

Two terms that have become popular in education are "prescriptive" and "diagnostic" teaching. These terms refer to a vital need in classroom instruction. Unless teaching techniques meet actual student needs, valuable time and energy are wasted, so far as educational growth is concerned.

This principle can be expressed another way in a three-point guide for practicality:

1. What does the student need?
2. What would be nice for him to know?
3. What is irrelevant at this time?

In correcting dyslexia in the classroom, this simplified statement is of great importance. If Mike does not know the alphabet, then this is his *need* of the moment. It would be *nice* for him to read twenty-five books this year. It would be totally *irrelevant* for him to attempt to write book reports. In other words, if the foundation has never been laid, it is foolish to attempt to build the upper floors. If the child needs the foundation, regardless of his chronological age or number of years in school, then the foundation is where the teacher must begin.

Because dyslexics have not fitted the standard academic mold, they are termed "disabled." When classroom teachers discover each student's need, as differentiated from the nice and the irrelevant, then a prescription can be drawn up specifying exact skills or knowledge the student has failed to perceive. This practical approach is simple, direct, and nontheoretical. By filling the student's need, the teacher enables him to move on to the things it would be nice for him to know. As needs are fulfilled, the formerly irrelevant areas become increasingly relevant. Teachers find themselves constructing the higher level skills surprisingly soon, once a solid foundation has been laid.

Principle 3: Relax the Pressure

The dyslexic student has two mortal enemies: a rapid work rate and pressure for quantity. As described in earlier chapters, dyslexics must work extremely slowly as they encode and decode. There simply is no way to hurry the process of translating language symbols that continually rotate, turn upside down, or otherwise refuse to remain fixed in the reader's perception. One of the deadliest experiences for the dyslexic is to be threatened by speed in a reading or writing situation. A universally expressed emotion in dyslexics is panic, particularly when they are forced to work under timed limitations. Rigidly timed standardized tests are especially threatening to most dyslexics. The click of a stopwatch or the crunching arm of a timing clock spells doom for these handicapped performers. Time penalties are as cruel for dyslexics as being forced to run in a track meet would be for a child with a withered leg. Teachers who are unaware of this reaction to time pressure can inflict damaging trauma in these students whose reactions are necessarily slow when processing symbols.

Pressure for quantity is equally devastating for dyslexic students. When confronted by assignments which specify considerable productivity within a limited amount of time, dyslexics invariably give up. A major cause of discipline problems in school is that too much quantity is expected from handicapped students. As pointed out in earlier chapters, dyslexics work many times more slowly than others. A rule of thumb for the classroom teacher would be to expect dyslexic students to work five to ten times more slowly than students without handicaps. This means that, if typical youngsters can do twenty problems in half an hour, dyslexics would generally do well to complete four or five problems in the same length of time. If most students in the class can handle five pages of silent reading during a study period, the dyslexic reader would do well to cover one page by himself.

When teachers can allow for these very real limitations in work rate, dyslexics usually prove willing to do their best. When handicapped students realize they are being dealt with according to their needs, they tend to respond positively. If given ample time to complete their work, dyslexic students are often the hardest workers in the class. If the purpose of assignments is to strengthen skills, then it does not matter whether conscientious students do five or twenty exercises, so long as each class member does his best. Teachers set their students up for failure when quantity, rather than quality, becomes the goal.

In dealing with dyslexic learners, the classroom teacher may occasionally be placed on the defensive, particularly when productivity is determined on a relative basis according to individual student needs. However, when educators really believe that every child is entitled to an education according to his needs, ways can be devised to fill those needs. To allow dyslexic children to fail just to pacify critical students, parents, or colleagues is difficult to defend. Relaxing pressures for speed and quantity is a reasonable educational objective, particularly for students who are incapable of fulfilling traditional expectations.

Principle 4: Keep It Simple

There is nothing simple about today's elementary curriculum. Brilliant adults who delight in manipulating complicated theory sets have designed "modern math," the "new English," and advanced science programs for elementary schools. Each new textbook adoption startles teachers who see difficult concepts being brought into primary and kindergarten education. Pressure is exerted for cramming more and more into the already complex school day of most children. This buildup of high expectations is lethal for perceptually impaired youngsters who are only confused by the bombardment of stimuli encountered at every turn. Even fun time is so overorganized in many schools that sensitive children dread recess.

Dyslexia involves the inability to sort out sensory impressions satisfactorily. New theories of learning indicate that classroom success is probably not a matter of learning how to react appropriately to certain stimuli. Instead, academic achievement may be the result of learning how *not* to react to the countless peripheral stimuli which bombard us from every side. The dyslexic child is unable to tune out irrelevant stimuli. He cannot edit his environment to identify what is relevant. When confronted by several stimuli at the same time, the dyslexic is unable to filter out those that are nonessential. Consequently his perception is inaccurate, leaving him unable to cope with the complicated learning expectations of today's curriculum.

Dyslexia can be remediated only when learning tasks present the child with controlled stimulus factors. This means that remediation of dyslexia calls for simple, step-by-step routines involving the student in only the amount of stimulus he can handle at a given time. Multiple stimuli seem to cancel each other out. For example, when lessons or study activities include several factors, the dyslexic student is overstimulated. Because he cannot cope with a variety of expectations at the same time, he fails to comprehend. The result is either neutral (no gain) or negative (loss). If, however, dyslexics are guided from one skill to the next at a pace they can handle, eventually they learn to cope with complicated tasks. Classroom teachers who are able to control the stimulus ingredients of their presentations find dyslexic children making surprising progress.

Since the principle of simplicity has always been at the heart of good teaching, curriculum materials are usually programmed to introduce discrete factors step by step. The problem is not so much with materials or with curriculum goals. The problem is in trying to accomplish too much too quickly. Dyslexics face crushing defeat when they are pressured to hurry through myriad skill levels before each level has become habitual or automatic. It is imperative that teachers keep their instruction simple until perceptual foundations are firmly laid in handicapped students.

Principle 5: Keep It Structured

No one has estimated the ratio of discoverers to nondiscoverers in our population. Classroom teachers are confronted by curriculum goals based on the premise that children "will" discover fundamental concepts through appropriate exploratory activities. Few would deny the impressive arguments of educationists that many children can be led to discover principles and laws if provided sufficient opportunities to explore. Perhaps the difficulty lies in translating learning theory into workable commercial programs used by everyday classroom teachers. The fact is that millions of American children are not learning computation, grammar, science, or reading in spite of superb materials and competent leadership.

A cardinal truth regarding perceptual impairment is that the learning of skills must be highly structured, as a rule. This principle does not actually contradict modern theories of self-discovery. The fact is that certain children cannot cope with loosely structured situations. Divergent thinking simply is not possible for many children until they have experienced specific, limited drill in foundation skills. Dyslexics cannot assemble parts into coherent wholes unless there is a clearly defined model in view. Abstract reasoning without visible structure is a major stumbling block for the perceptually impaired.

Classroom teachers are faced with the need to insure structured, regular teaching routines upon which dyslexic learners can depend. This rules out certain kinds of multiple stimulus activities specified in teachers' manuals and guidebooks. A critical need of disabled learners is for structured guidelines which hold their form. Words with multiple meanings, variant spellings of vowel or consonant sounds, open-ended grammar or punctuation rules, and indefinite elements of math, science, and social studies all appear threatening to children who cannot function without dependable visual-auditory-tactile cues.

Classroom Activities for Visual Dyslexics

Establishing Sequence

As described in Chapters 1 and 2, failure to comprehend sequence is a major handicap of visual dyslexics. This tendency is aggravated by the assumptions of adults that cultural factors involving sequence or seriation are as obvious to children as to grown-ups. Few teachers have ever analyzed their own habits or mannerisms when giving instructions. It would astonish most teachers to discover how really fuzzy and out of focus their classroom directions often appear to students. Children usually succeed because they second-guess adults well, not because the instructions have been very clear.

Teaching Chronological Sequence.   The first step in establishing awareness of time sequence is to provide children with visible, tangible cue systems that illustrate chronological order. In primary grades this is usually done with monthly calendars to establish the days of the week within the month. Few teachers present time in more than thirty-day calendar units.

Dyslexic children must be drilled in the basic units of time: seconds and minutes; minutes and hours; hours and days; days and weeks; weeks and months; months and years; and years and centuries. Busy teachers usually bypass steps in this continuum, hopping from minutes and hours to days and weeks, omitting years and centuries altogether. Primary activities seldom build an unbroken, sequential awareness of time, showing the continuum from the smallest units (seconds) to largest units (centuries). Bright children without dyslexic tendencies soon deduce this sort of time structure in our culture. But, without visible, tangible models as constant reminders, dyslexics fail to perceive the order and segmentation of time. This has crippling results in social studies (historical sequence), math (lapse of time), and science (seasonal change; geological classification). This basic deficit in time sequence leaves the dyslexic unable to cope with many curriculum expectations which adults take for granted.

Every classroom should have tangible charts illustrating progressive time relationships, which should be displayed in sequence all year long. Dyslexic students need to be involved in daily renewal of their awareness of time units. Other students who have already grasped the concepts should not be dragged through irrelevant repetitions. But children who have not yet mastered sequence should be reviewed consistently until all of it begins to fall into place.

In September school should begin with a visual model of how summer has merged into fall. Day by day the pupils should see a visual progression involving such concepts as these: during last summer; this fall; when winter comes; last week; now; next week; last month (August); this month (September); next month (October); how long until Christmas (December), and so on. Much of the time that teachers spend fashioning bulletin board displays to keep the room interesting should be devoted to a permanent, step-by-step presentation of time sequence, in which nothing is left to chance. When this sort of carefully programmed sequence of time is done, teachers see dyslexic youngsters beginning to grasp the concepts of chronological order. As birthdays and other personal events are incorporated into the visual time model, children begin to comprehend this aspect of seriation in our culture.

Creative teachers will have no difficulty turning one wall of their classrooms into an effective, colorful time map for dyslexic pupils. The great temptation is for teachers to go back to their old habits of neglecting this sort of perceptual training in order to "get through the books on schedule." Getting through the books is irrelevant for students who still have not mastered sequence. If teachers can understand that some children will more than make up the pages in the books *after* the foundation has been laid, then the importance of daily attention to building concepts of time sequence will be easier to live with in the classroom.

At this point it is essential to ask: "What do these children need?" If they need daily instruction in the fundamentals of chronological order, then getting through unit 2 of science or social studies is irrelevant. There is nothing shameful about rote drill to master the days of the week or the months of the year in chronological order. The ultimate goal of such drill is comprehension of how specific days and months fit into the serial order of the calendar. Before this level of practical understanding can be reached, however, dyslexics must spend many hours of drilling to name the days and months, as well as to write them from memory. It is a serious cultural deficit for an individual in the labor market to stumble over which day it is, or which month. Instead of belaboring her handicapped students over irrelevant textbook matter, the teacher should spend their time establishing a solid working knowledge of time sequence, regardless of the age of the students involved.

Teaching Alphabetic Sequence.   For forty years American educators have thought themselves astute for concealing alphabetic sequence until after children have learned to read. For most children this has done no harm, largely because these youngsters have been learning the alphabet anyway from model cards displayed in primary classrooms. Dyslexic children have been left out in the cold because of their inability to comprehend sequence presented in an indirect way. Because they have not perceived positional relationships between discrete letter forms, these handicapped students are stymied when called upon to alphabetize words, find entries in the dictionary, or locate material in reference books. When letter forms are doled out in random order, there is no point of reference by which the dyslexic child can comprehend the relative positions of letters within the alphabetic sequence. This deficiency poses serious problems for independent study in upper grades.

Teachers of dyslexics must recover from the guilt feelings engendered by professors of education who have taught that rote drill is questionable, to say the least. Dyslexic children have no other choice by virtue of their handicap. If alphabetic sequence is to be mastered, it must be done through rote drill—day after day of toil, arranging movable letter forms in correct order, copying from clear models, and writing the sequence from memory. If the child *needs* to learn alphabetic sequence, then it is irrelevant for him to struggle through higher level activities which rest upon such knowledge.

Beginner pupils should start learning alphabetic sequence by manipulating three-dimensional forms. Many kinds of commercial letter sets are on the market, ranging from inexpensive cardboard to costly kits of lacquered wood. Creative teachers can devise their own alphabet models using clay, pipe cleaners, or hand-cut paper forms. It is totally unnecessary for a school to spend precious funds on expensive materials to teach alphabetic sequence. In fact, the simpler the models, the better they usually are for teaching purposes in the classroom.

In mastering the alphabet, it is essential that dyslexic children learn only one major concept at a time. For this reason it is detrimental for a teacher to introduce phonic principles at the same time letter shapes are being mastered. Dyslexic children must not be expected to manipulate two forms of information at once while in the initial stages of acquiring a perceptual foundation. For example, Mike should associate the *names* of the letters with their shapes, not the sounds which the letter forms represent. He should match the letter A with the name of the letter, but he should not be exposed to "phonics" until he has first learned to associate the letter name with its form. Sounds for symbols should come *after* sequence and forms of symbols have been mastered.

Alert teachers will be able to tell when a child is ready for a more advanced level of experience in handling alphabetic sequence. The following increment scale suggests the kinds of sequential activities the teacher can monitor in the classroom.

Step One	Master alphabetic sequence with movable letter forms (sandpaper letters, if this learning is difficult for the child)
Step Two	Trace over alphabetic sequence on chalkboard
Step Three	Trace over alphabetic sequence on paper (or on plastic wipe-off alphabet sheets)
Step Four	Copy alphabetic sequence on chalkboard (by following model cards or teacher's written model)
Step Five	Copy alphabetic sequence on lined paper (following chart model or teacher's written model)
Step Six	Write alphabetic sequence with visual model in view (to check against reversals or transpositions)
Step Seven	Write alphabetic sequence from memory with no reversals, rotations, or letters out of sequence

The mistake teachers have made is rushing children too fast through this developmental sequence. Today's kindergarten programs usually introduce Step One and Step Two. Most schools assume that primary pupils have mastered all seven steps by beginning Grade Three. This is not the case, as revealed by thousands of high school students who cannot handle alphabetic sequence from memory. The urgent need of the dyslexic is that this educational need be fulfilled, no matter how old the student is when the deficiency is discovered. It is irrelevant for students to struggle with book reports or themes until they have mastered the sequence of the alphabet.

Traditionally, cursive writing style has been postponed until Grade Three on the assumption that primary children need to learn the gross motor skills of acceptable manuscript print before advancing to the more complicated motor patterns of cursive style. This assumption has never been effectively supported by research evidence. On the contrary, children who begin handwriting with cursive style seldom manifest disabling dysgraphic tendencies in later writing activities. Largely because of the consistent, flowing motor patterns established through cursive writing, alphabetic sequence is quickly established when cursive style is introduced.

The quickest remediation of reversal and rotation tendencies in writing is quite simple. The teacher writes a clearly legible line of alphabet letters, all connected in cursive style as if she were spelling one long word. Then the child practices tracing over the written model as the teacher guides his wrist to establish proper hand movements. Over a period of a few weeks this kind of practice pays off generously. The dyslexic child becomes increasingly self-confident at writing. His perception of alphabetic sequence quickly develops, and he becomes aware of the relative positions of letters within the sequence. By having a dependable model as a guide, visual dyslexics find great security. Soon they are ready to progress to copying the teacher's handwriting directly beneath her written model. In a few days or weeks the children can write their own cursive sequence with only occasional reference to a model. For dysgraphic children, described in Chapter 4, the process of remediation is slow and frustrating. Cursive writing style is, however, the most directly feasible avenue to establishing automatic knowledge of alphabetic sequence.

Comprehending Instructions. Faulty comprehension of time and alphabetic sequence is largely a personal problem, involving the dyslexic learner with private failure in specific classroom assignments. The inability to comprehend instructions widens the area of conflict to include classmates and family members. When dyslexics fail to observe the teacher's intentions regarding assigned activities, the whole group is ultimately involved in the disrupted classroom atmosphere.

Helping children attend to sequential steps in carrying out classroom expectations is actually rather simple. Instead of forcing children to depend upon memory, the teacher must provide a simple encoded outline of her expectations. If the students can read, this is accomplished by listing sequential steps on a chart or the chalkboard. This technique is especially suitable for routine work, such as classroom chores or daily work schedules which remain fairly constant from day to day. When a clear instructional sequence is provided in the child's text or workbooks, the teacher has a ready-made visual aid in teaching how to follow sequence in interpreting instructions. Otherwise the teacher must make her own visual models around the room.

Kindergarten and primary teachers often solve the problem by creating nonverbal code systems, such as using animal pictures, colored shapes, or other easily decoded symbol sets as cues. Children who lose track easily can refer to the chart to be reminded of what to do next.

Older dyslexics have the same basic needs for quick reference. As they listen to a series of directions, dyslexics immediately lose the sequence of expectations. Most teachers are unaware of how complicated their oral directions actually are. For example, in getting her arithmetic class underway, a teacher in Grade Four will usually make twenty or more discrete statements. Children are adept at "tuning in" and "tuning out" so they seldom attend to all the teacher says. They are expected to "filter" the teacher's dialogue.

A transcript of this kind of situation might read as follows:

> Now, children, it's time for arithmetic. Put away your social studies books and get out your arithmetic books. Tom, sit down. Yes, Mary? No, you don't need two pencils. Now, class, be sure you have your pencils ready. Open your workbooks to today's lesson. Yes, Joe? No, I didn't *say* get them out, but you know I meant for you to. Now, children, open your books to page 251. What, Sue? Yes, you may get a drink for your hiccups. Now, on page 251 we are ready to review short division. . . .

This steady flow of dialogue is supplemented by paralanguage, the unspoken gestures, facial expressions, variations of tone, and myriad other ingredients of group communication. Most children edit the running dialogue, tuning in only when the teacher or a fellow student utters a relevant statement or command. A student without a handicap would monitor the teacher's dialogue like this:

> . . . it's time for arithmetic. . . . Put away your social studies books . . . get out your arithmetic books . . . you don't need two pencils . . . open your workbooks to today's lesson . . . open your books to page 251 . . . we are ready to review short division. . . .

The dyslexic listener cannot edit successfully. He is unable to determine what the teacher thinks essential because he cannot filter out the extraneous peripheral stimuli bombarding him from all sides. When there is no visual cue to outline the essential tasks for him, the dyslexic is lost. However, if his teacher has provided a tangible model for later reference, the student has a chance. By referring to the following outline on the chalkboard, he can cope with the teacher's expectations:

For Today's Arithmetic
1. Have one pencil ready.
2. Open textbook to page 251.
3. Open workbook to page 97.
4. For tomorrow do the 15 problems on workbook page 97.

Many teachers have found it expedient to tape record their daily instructions. After the class is at work, those who did not comprehend the instructions can slip on headphones and listen to the assignment in private, repeating the instructions as many times as needed. As a last resort, they can go to the teacher individually. When some kind of face-saving alternative is provided for dyslexics, the entire group is spared the agonies encountered when one or two students disrupt the learning atmosphere by clamoring for repeated explanations.

Failure to comprehend sequence in instructions is the primary cause for failure with arithmetic story problems, science experiments, and chronological order in social studies. Although outlining is often introduced in elementary grades, the purpose for making brief outlines is frequently not clear to the students. An essential skill for the dyslexic is being able to put down the essential ingredients of a problem step by step. Providing instruction charts or tapes is one way of outlining what the adult expects of the child. Leaving the interpretation of commands up to the student is not fair, unless the teacher has taken great pains to insure clarity. The overwhelming need of dyslexics is for the adult to leave easily retraceable steps for them to follow. If the handicapped student has easily deciphered cues, he can learn to cope with most classroom expectations.

Correcting Reversals and Rotations

Teaching visual dyslexics not to turn elements upside down or backwards is not always possible in a typical classroom setting. This tendency usually requires a one-to-one teaching relationship which few teachers can provide during the school day. There are certain remedial steps, however, which can be taken regardless of the teacher's time limitations.

Remediation must begin with honesty. This statement may seem strange to many seasoned educators who are above reproach in their personal ethics. Teachers, however, seldom deal forthrightly with problems involving perceptual impairment. If a student is to find relief from lifelong tendencies toward disability, these must be dealt with openly and forthrightly. This does not mean that an adult would place a student in a position of embarrassment or chagrin before his peers. The approach required for successful remedial work with dyslexics in the classroom is that of informing the student of the kinds of mistakes he tends to make, and then developing a cue system to help him monitor his work against such mistakes in the future.

In a quiet conference away from the prying eyes and ears of other students, the teacher should explain how the handicapped child's work has been analyzed for dyslexic characteristics. For example, the teacher should present a checklist of visual dyslexic characteristics (see end of Chapter 2). This tangible list of deficiencies helps her explain in simple terms that the child does not "see" letters, numerals, or words like most people do. Many professionals recoil from this sort of counseling on the grounds that it is cruel and dangerous to expose a child to himself. The fact is that it is cruel *not* to explain to the handicapped person exactly what it is that produces conflict in his learning situation. Of course it would be foolish in most instances to tell a child, "Mike, you are dyslexic." If Mike is mature enough to ask specifically what his problem is, however, he should be told. Half the success of remediating these tendencies depends upon the child's full cooperation. It is impossible to enlist the student's cooperation if he is not informed of the nature of the problems he is supposed to be correcting.

A teacher will readily understand the need for honesty by recalling how she feels when medical doctors withhold information about her own illnesses. Adults are quickly frightened when an examining physician mutters "Hmmmmm!" to himself, or "Aha!" but never explains all of this to the apprehensive patient. If teachers can realize that children have the same needs for clarity as adults, it will make remedial work with dyslexics a great deal more effective.

Quietly, unemotionally, and forthrightly the teacher should point to specific examples of dyslexic confusion in the child's work, explaining that these are the reasons for low grades or other forms of failure. The child should be told that he "sees some letters backwards or upside down," and the teacher should point out exact instances in his work (*beb* for bed; *mnst* for must). Or she might play part of a tape to let the student hear himself invert syllables ("gril" for girl; "on" for no). Whatever the dyslexic tendencies are, the teacher must explain them to the student, in whatever detail the student wishes. The teacher must not be judgmental or condescending. If the conference can be conducted as a conversation between an interested adult and a child with a need, the result will be relief and a sense of understanding on the child's part. After all, he has known for a long time that something has been wrong. At last somebody is explaining it all to him.

Teachers should allow the dyslexic to suggest ways for correcting the problem, especially in upper grades. Particularly intelligent primary pupils are usually able to have a voice in planning their remedial activities. The teacher must make it clear what her expectations are. This is often done in the form of a simple contract which states the specific dyslexic problems and what the child promises to do each day to overcome them. The teacher must make it clear how much time she can give in individual tutoring during the school day. If she can manage three five-minute periods during recess periods or the lunch hour, this needs to be specified. The important thing is that the student know how much individual attention he can expect.

The most promising source of help for one-to-one tutoring during the school day is older students, volunteer teacher aides, or other individuals who can fit quietly into the school routine without disrupting classroom procedures. Older students are especially effective as tutors, provided there is no clash between them and the dyslexic child. A small amount of attention on a one-to-one basis goes a long way in building self-confidence in the dyslexic. Tutoring need not go on for hours to be effective. In fact, three thirty-minute sessions during the school week are often enough to unlock the perceptual block, allowing the dyslexic student to make significant progress in overcoming his handicap.

Arithmetic. Chapter 1 discusses briefly the perceptual dilemma dyslexic children face in mastering arithmetic skills. The major deficit is inability to change direction without becoming confused and losing the mental picture of the number relationships involved. Arithmetic computation above the primary level involves thousands of transformations as sets, number units, and abstractions change positions within problem forms. Arithmetic symbols represent highly condensed decoding (reading). A single symbol often stands for a complex abstract concept. It would take many lines of prose to express clearly the memory factors involved in most simple appearing problems and equations. Students who tend to scramble sequence, lose directionality, and reverse and transpose entities within patterns find it very difficult to master the myriad variations they encounter beyond beginning computation levels.

The foremost consideration for teachers to keep in mind when working with dyslexics is to keep the structure as nearly the same as possible. It is distressing for dyslexics to have to shift back and forth from linear form $7 + \underline{} = 13$ to vertical form

$$\begin{array}{r} 7. \\ + \\ \hline 13 \end{array}$$

Lessons requiring students to transform rapidly or frequently impose so much memory stress that most dyslexics quickly become agitated or rebellious.

Wise teachers who recognize memory and directional problems in their students keep the format of problems the same. Dyslexics are capable of learning linear form (equations), but they cannot rapidly change back and forth from one mode to another. Since the goal of education is to prepare students for future situations beyond the classroom, it is totally unimportant that all children change directionality quickly on demand, just for practice. Dyslexics need structure which stays the same as much of the time as possible. Whenever teachers must vary the problem form, dyslexic students must be given time and help in making the perceptual change. Some children never learn to do so at all. For them, the standard vertical problem mode is essential since this is the style they will need the most in their future private lives.

An increasingly common practice is to let children use inexpensive pocket calculators for classroom computing. Dyslexics need to develop functional knowledge of paper/pencil computing, of course, but there is no way they can handle the quantity of work prescribed by most classroom programs. Mike cannot possibly work arithmetic problems faster than his usual plodding rate. Of necessity his work is labored and prolonged when he must translate mental images into written forms. A hand calculator gives him an instant means of speeding up his work, and the increase in his self-confidence is just as rapid. With a calculator he can pour out arithmetic work along with the fastest pencil performers in the class. What a boost to his morale it is to hold his own after so much embarrassment and sense of failure.

High school and college math instructors are making wide use of pocket calculators. In fact, the slide rule in math courses is becoming obsolete. Forcing disabled students to labor with traditional paper/pencil computation is just as obsolete, especially when no real purpose is served except for satisfying tradition. "We've always done it this way" does not justify forcing dyslexics to agonize over memorized facts when a remarkably simple new form is now available. The pocket calculator has come into its own as a valid educational tool. Teachers who resist its use are refusing to step into the twentieth century.

A wide variety of publications now offers classroom techniques for teaching arithmetic skills to dyslexics (see reading list at the end of this chapter).* Watchful teachers will discover a wide variety of new materials appearing as more attention is given to teaching arithmetic to children with special needs.

Classroom teachers must keep two cardinal rules in mind when teaching arithmetic skills to dyslexic children:

1. Keep the structure constant

Because conservation of form (reversibility and transformation) is so difficult for dyslexics, arithmetic structure must remain the same from day to day. Frequent changes in mode, format, and directionality are devastating to confused students who cannot handle rapid shifts in form.

2. Keep the work rate slow

Dyslexics must not be pressured to hurry in computation. If quantity is important, then they must be given the by-pass mode of a pocket calculator. A hand calculator is an equalizer, making up the vast difference between the perceptual endowments of rapid learners and the disabilities for which the dyslexic child is not responsible. If paper/pencil routines are essential, then the work rate must be slow. If calculators are permitted, then the dyslexic can produce as much arithmetic work as his peers.

Reading Orally. Reading aloud is a prime avenue for correcting reversals and rotations. As the dyslexic child reads slowly from one text, his tutor monitors from another copy. As mistakes occur, the monitor quietly says, "Look at that word again, Mike; how is it spelled?" This sort of cueing is low key. There is no embarrassment or shame in calling the child's attention to his errors. By immediately pinpointing error patterns, the tutor reinforces accurate symbol perception on a one-to-one basis. The intelligent dyslexic soon begins to catch his own errors by coordinating what he sees, says, and hears.

Using Tachistoscopes. Individual perceptual training is augmented through the use of tachistoscopes of various kinds. These devices range from simple handmade flash cards to expensive electronic instruments mounted in learning booths. An inexpensive commercial instrument that is highly effective in developing accurate word recognition is the Flash X, marketed by EDL (Educational Developmental Laboratories, Inc.). For less than twenty dollars two or three Flash X units with appropriate

---

* Especially helpful are two paperback anthologies published by Academic Therapy Publications, 1539 Fourth Street, San Rafael, California 94901: *Building Arithmetic Skills in Dyslexic Children* and *These Kids Don't Count.*

word cards can be purchased. The dyslexic student practices perceiving whole word units in a fraction of a second. He immediately tries to pronounce the word, and then he writes it quickly while the visual image is still fresh. Finally he opens a shutter to check his work for accuracy. This kind of forced response is highly effective in correcting faulty perception, particularly when reversal and rotation tendencies are involved.

Matching Word Forms. Daily drill activities can be devised by the monitor or teacher to develop accuracy in word discrimination. A simple word is presented on a flash card. After a quick glance, the dyslexic student tries to find a matching word within a line of similar word forms. The following examples from the JWST (see Appendix B) illustrate how this can be done in the classroom.

barn	bran	pran	puar	buar	narb	uarp	barn
spot	spot	tobs	tops	stop	stob	sbot	tobs
silver	sliver	silver	vilser	rivils	revlis	selvir

Keeping Track of Progress

Those teachers who conquer dyslexia in the classroom usually keep track of progress. This should be a simple procedure, requiring a minimum of bookkeeping. Older children can learn to record their own progress, as they do in other individualized study programs utilized by many schools. The initial task is for the teacher to prepare a guide sheet, outlining the child's specific dyslexic tendencies. The checklist used for diagnosis is a convenient basis for constructing the guide sheet. Brief comments should be recorded to indicate improvement. The final entry beside each dyslexic characteristic is the date when the problem has come under control. Of course it is impossible to know the very day when certain tendencies disappear. But the child and his tutor can compile a record of improvement, which is the major consideration in building self-confidence. This simple diagnostic record offers two advantages for remedial work in the classroom. First, prescriptive teaching is quite simple, once the specific deficiencies have been identified on the checklist. This means that the teacher can pace the child's progress from one skill level to the next without undue frustration. Until the record sheet shows that specific problems have been cleared up, the teacher knows not to push the child on to a more frustrating level of activity. Second, the record sheet forms the basis for a reasonable work contract between the child and his tutor. The dyslexic student knows exactly how much remains to be remediated in his learning behavior. Without this simple record and communication between teacher and child, everyone involved continues to wallow in frustration and failure.

The dyslexic child's frustration threshold is an accurate index to the success of remedial activities. So long as the tutor observes tension, disruptive behavior, frustration, anxiety, dread, avoidance tactics, and other symptoms of learning difficulty, she knows the child's learning disabilities remain operational. Regardless of the age of the student or the lateness in the year, it is useless and dangerous to push the dyslexic student further and further on through the books. The teacher will know when the perceptual foundation has taken hold. The child will begin to exhibit long-range tranquillity in comparison to his former frustrated behavior during study activities. When the student can work rather calmly for long periods of time (half an hour or more) with materials which used to bring disruptive reactions, the teacher will know that remediation has been effective. Then it will be time to take the child to the next step of perceptual development.

Making Referrals

Four out of five dyslexics in the classroom can respond to the techniques suggested in this chapter. Some cannot. Approximately twenty percent of the handicapped students require specialized remedial therapy away from a group environment. Teachers should call for help when it is indicated. However, classroom teachers must not give up on a child because of the convenience of having him placed elsewhere.

Unfortunately, only a handful of clinics and other institutions specialize in dyslexia. Many reading clinics do not deal with this disability. In fact, some clinical services deny that such a reading disability exists. A rule of thumb for referral to other agencies might be this:

> So long as the child is making some progress, I'll keep up my efforts to cope with his problems in my classroom. When his behavior becomes so disruptive that others cannot learn or when he becomes so frustrated he cannot continue in a group, then I'll refer him to another agency for special help.

If there is no outside help available for seriously dyslexic students, the classroom teacher can make a trustworthy diagnosis by using the instruments and techniques presented in this book. Many communities are forming volunteer helping-hands groups of interested parents, teenagers, or college students to take some pressure off the disabled students in local classrooms. Churches, civic organizations, and the PTA are potential allies of the classroom teacher, once such volunteer groups are shown that the need exists.

References for Further Reading

1. Abrams, J. C. "Further Considerations on the Ego Functioning of the Dyslexic Child—A Psychiatric Viewpoint." *Reading Disability and Perception.* Newark, Delaware: International Reading Association, Proceedings of the 13th Annual Convention, vol. 13, part 3 (1969): 16-21.

2. Adelman, H. S. "Learning Problems, Part II: A Sequential and Hierarchial Approach to Identification and Correction. *Academic Therapy Quarterly* 6 (Spring 1971): 287-292.

3. Applegate, Ellen. *Perceptual Aids in the Classroom.* San Rafael, California. Academic Therapy Publications, 1968.

4. Auxter, David. "Reaction Time of Children with Learning Disabilities." *Academic Therapy Quarterly* 6 (Winter 1970-71): 151-154.

5. Behrmann, Polly. *Activities for Developing Visual-Perception.* San Rafael, California: Academic Therapy Publications, 1970.

6. Benyon, S. D. *Intensive Programming for Slow Learners.* Columbus, Ohio: Charles E. Merrill Publishing Co., 1968.

7. Bryant, N. D. "Some Principles of Remedial Instruction for Dyslexia." *Children with Reading Problems.* Edited by Gladys Natchez, pp. 397-403. New York: Basic Books, 1968.

8. Copeland, R. W. *Diagnostic and Learning Activities in Mathematics for Children.* New York: MacMillan Publishing Co., 1974.

9. Cratty, Bryant J. *Active Learning: Games to Enhance Academic Abilities.* pp. 47-77. Englewood Cliffs: Prentice-Hall, Inc., 1971.

10. Davis, J. H., and Edgington, Ruth. "Classroom Teaching Suggestions for Language-Learning Problems." *Academic Therapy Quarterly* 5 (Fall 1969): 67-74.

11. Dubnoff, Belle. "Building Ego Factors through the Curriculum." *Journal of Learning Disabilities* 3 (September 1970): 459-466.

12. Early, G. H. "Developing Perceptual-Motor Skills: Integrating the Perceptual Modalities." *Academic Therapy Quarterly* 5 (Winter 1969-70): 133-136.

13. Emrick, C. D. "Treatment of Conceptual and Perceptual Deficits." *Academic Therapy Quarterly* 6 (Spring 1971): 293-303.

14. Felton, Sandra, *et al.* "A Multiplication Process." *Academic Therapy Quarterly* 9 (Winter 1973-74): 249-251.

15. Fogerty, Lucile L. "Mathematics in the Primary Grades." *Teaching Educationally Handicapped Children.* Edited by John I. Arena. pp. 71-74. San Rafael, California: Academic Therapy Publications, 1967.

16. Frostig, Marianne. "Disabilities and Remediation in Reading." *Academic Therapy Quarterly* 7 (Summer 1972): 373-391.

17. Glavach, Matt, and Stoner, Donovan. "Breaking the Failure Pattern." *Journal of Learning Disabilities* 3 (February 1970): 103-105.

18. Griffiths, A. N. "Self-Concept in Remedial Work with Dyslexic Children." *Academic Therapy Quarterly* 6 (Winter 1970-71): 125-133.

19. Haskell, Simon H. *Arithmetical Disabilities in Cerebral Palsied Children: Programmed Instruction—A Remedial Approach.* London: University of London, 1973.

20. Isgur, Jay. "Establishing Letter-Sound Associations by an Object-Imaging-Projection Method." *Journal of Learning Disabilities* 8 (June/July 1975): 349-353.

21. Johnson, D. J. "Treatment Approaches to Dyslexia." *Reading Disability and Perception.* Newark, Delaware: International Reading Association, Proceedings of the 13th Annual Convention, vol. 13, part 3 (1969): 95-102.

22. Karlin, Muriel S., and Berger, Regina. *Successful Methods for Teaching the Slow Learner.* West Nyack, N.Y.: Parker Publishing Company, Inc., 1969.

23. *Mathematics Learning in Early Childhood: 37th Yearbook.* Reston, Va.: National Council of Teachers of Mathematics, 1975.

24. Miller, Julano. "Skill Checklist." *Academic Therapy Quarterly* 11 (Winter 1975-76): 243-249.

25. Mitchell, Elizabeth. *Ideas for Teaching Inefficient Learners.* San Rafael, Calif.: Academic Therapy Publications, 1968.

26. Murphy, Patricia. "Teach with a Wooden Clown: Perceptual Techniques and Materials." *Meeting the Needs of Dyslexic Children and Others.* Reprint Collection no. 2. San Rafael, Calif.: Academic Therapy Publications (1969): 39-44.

27. Myers, P. I., and Hammill, D. D. *Methods for Learning Disorders.* New York: John Wiley & Sons, 1969.

28. Orton, J. L. "The Orton-Gillingham Approach." *The Disabled Reader: Education of the Dyslexic Child.* Edited by John Money, pp. 119-145. Baltimore: The Johns Hopkins Press, 1966.

29. Peskin, Anne, and Tauber-Scheidlinger, Roselyn. "Let Them Learn Their Way." *Academic Therapy Quarterly* 11 (Spring 1976) 301-311.

30. Peterson, D. *Functional Mathematics for the Mentally Retarded.* Columbus, Ohio: Charles E. Merrill Publishing Company, 1973.

31. Rosner, Jerome. *Two Developmental Training Devices.* San Rafael, Calif.: Academic Therapy Publications, 1971.

32. Savage, E. V. "Suggested Approaches to Overcoming Reversals in Reading." *Meeting the Needs of Dyslexic Children, and Others.* Reprint Collection no. 2. San Rafael, Calif.: Academic Therapy and Publications (1969): 8-10.

33. Scheffelin, Margaret A., and Seltzer, Carl. "Math Manipulations for Learning Disabilities." *Academic Therapy Quarterly* 9 (Spring 1974): 357-362.

34. Sharp, Eunice. "Creativity in Arithmetic for Educationally Handicapped Children. *"Teaching Educationally Handicapped Children.* Edited by John I. Arena, pp. 67-70. San Rafael, Calif.: Academic Therapy Publications, 1967.

35. Shoemaker, Linda C. "Learning to Remember." *Academic Therapy Quarterly* 7 (Winter 1971-72): 227-235.

36. Sklar, B., and Henley, J. "A Multi-Fontal Alphabet for Dyslexic Children." *Journal of Learning Disabilities* 5 (March 1972): 160-164.

37. Smith, Deborah D., and Lovitt, Thomas C. "The Differential Effects of Reinforcement Contingencies on Arithmetic Performance." *Journal of Learning Disabilities* 9 (January 1976): 32-40.

38. Solan, H. A. "Visual Processing Training with the Tachistoscope: A Rationale and Grade One Norms." *Journal of Learning Disabilities* 2 (January 1969): 30-36.

39. Stanberg, Les, and Mauser, August J. "The L.D. Child and Mathematics." *Academic Therapy Quarterly* 10 (Summer 1975): 481-488.

40. Wood, Mildred H. "Destructive Practices in Teaching Math." *Academic Therapy Quarterly* 10 (Winter 1974-75): 249-251.

41. Zach, Lillian, and Kaufman, Judith. "The Effect of Verbal Labelling on Visual Motor Performance." *Journal of Learning Disabilities* 2 (April 1969): 218-222.

chapter 6

Correcting Auditory Dyslexia in the Classroom

Since the advent of Dick and Jane, massive attention has been directed to the teaching of auditory skills, those skills which enable a child to identify specific elements of speech. Once the learner identifies the component sounds of oral language, it is theorized, he should have little difficulty in associating specific written symbols with discrete oral values. In other words, if a child "hears" speech sounds accurately, he should have no trouble making sound-symbol associations. Thus the student is expected to learn to encode the language he speaks and hears. The reverse process is decoding, or turning printed symbols into the oral language they represent.

On the surface this process of matching oral and written codes seems simple enough. After all, if the child will only listen, or attend, he can grasp the encoding and decoding processes through programmed routines which gradually lead him into higher level reading behaviors. Armed with this assumption, authors, publishers, and classroom teachers have created mountains of materials and techniques for teaching "auditory acuity," "auditory discrimination," "phonetic analysis," or just plain "phonics." To the frustration of the profession, however, a sizable minority of students do not master these skills, regardless of the hours spent on phonics drill.

Most children who do not develop auditory discrimination are dyslexics. Auditory dyslexia has been compared in Chapter 1 to tone deafness, meaning that the child does not notice differences between similar sounds in speech. This condition ranges from the inability to distinguish only two or three basic sounds to the inability to distinguish whole word units. Some children confuse only a few short vowel sounds. Others recognize no vowel distinctions at all. The problem is not difficulty with hearing (auding) as such. Instead, there is an inability to interpret correctly what is heard.

90

Although traditional phonics instruction teaches most children to decode efficiently, phonics drill, as it is usually presented in the elementary grades, is largely wasted on auditory dyslexics. If the tone-deaf dyslexic is to become a proficient reader and speller, different techniques must be used. Simply giving him a stringent diet of phonics usually does not solve the problem.

A major factor in auditory confusion is the way phonics is presented in most elementary reading circles. Only a few commercial reading programs begin reading instruction with carefully sequenced spelling patterns that follow the rules until the child is confident enough to handle variations from the rules. Beginner pupils are usually faced with a conglomeration of whole word units in which the sound-symbol relationships are variable and inconsistent. It is not uncommon for a primer story to contain several spellings of certain vowel or consonant sounds.

For example, an auditory dyslexic would be frustrated by the following reading experience:

> "Run, Sue!" called Mother. "Here are four cookies for you."
> "Good-bye, Bootsy," Sue said to her doll. "I will eat a cookie for you."

In spite of weeks of drill on individual phonemes (individual sound units), the dyslexic pupil is unable to cope with variant spellings of the same sound elements: run–Mother   Sue–to–you–Bootsy   for–four   I– Good–bye. He is equally confused by different sounds for the same letter groups: run–Sue   Here–her   cookies–Bootsy   you–four.

It is virtually meaningless to a dyslexic child to be told, "Listen for the long vowel sound in Sue. Do you hear *u* say its name?" Usually the dyslexic does not hear the vowel as distinguished from the consonant qualities. When the mysteries of decoding are presented in random order, the child with faulty auditory perception is lost from the start.

In seeking to remediate auditory dyslexia in the classroom, the teacher must keep certain principles in mind. Regardless of its attractiveness or success in other situations, a remedial technique cannot be effective unless the child's learning climate has been carefully established.

Principle 1: Make Immediate Tangible Applications of Abstract Rules

Generalizations about phonics are almost always taught in the abstract, even when the teacher thinks she is providing simple, concrete illustrations for her pupils. The teacher is dealing in abstractions when she shows the word *road* while emphasizing the "long sound of *o*." When shown the word configuration *road* and told, "Listen to *o* say its name," the child is confronted by three abstractions simultaneously: (1) the intellective act of attending to what the teacher says (tuning out extraneous peripheral stimuli); (2) the word form which represents the concept; and (3) the "sound of *o* saying its name." Because he is unable to isolate a specific stimulus from all the stimuli bombarding him, the dyslexic child cannot cope with even this simple cluster of oral/aural/ visual relationships. The result is lack of comprehension of what the teacher means. What appears to an adult to be a very simple learning exercise is to the dyslexic child a confusing jumble, a "roar," from which he gleans no specific meanings. Consequently, the child fails to please the teacher, and another experience in failure has transpired.

It is difficult for teachers to believe that older children, even high school students, may still need to work with concrete objects in order to nail down such foundation concepts as "Listen to *o* say its long name." Even dyslexic adults must experience kindergarten type of activities, such as manipulating movable letter forms, if they are to comprehend discrete sound values. If auditory dyslexics are to master the foundation concepts of sound-symbol relationships, they must experience immediate, tangible reinforcement. Teachers must realize that traditional reading circle practices have not worked with auditory dyslexics precisely because there is not enough concrete reinforcement of abstractions. Regardless of the student's age, it is usually necessary to provide concrete associative experiences between sounds and their symbol counterparts.

Principle 2: Provide Multisensory Experiences

Most teachers recall a concept from introductory psychology: The more senses involved in a learning experience, the more fully the experience is learned. This oversimplification of learning is a key to successful remediation of auditory dyslexia in the classroom. If a child sees it, hears it, says it, feels it, moves it—even smells it or tastes it—he can begin to comprehend it. In other words, the more sensory channels utilized by the teacher, the more comprehension attained by the pupils.

There is some risk involved in overanalyzing (sounding out), particularly when dealing with isolated sounds and symbols. Some children misperceive, resulting in grossly exaggerated sounding out of words that renders decoding impossible. For example, some children involved in current instructional programs that deal heavily with blending have the mistaken idea that each letter of the alphabet is a "word." *A* is "aye" or "aaaaaa," *B* is "bee" or "buh," *C* is "see" or "kuh," and so forth. It is perfectly natural, therefore, for such a child to perceive the word *cat* as three words, not three letters. Thus he would articulate: "cuh–aaaaaa–tuh." Because this is like nothing he hears in daily language usage, he completely misses the concept for which *cat* stands.

The risks involved in overanalyzing should not cause teachers to back away from multisensory teaching techniques. As a rule, the relatively few children who develop such grossly distorted concepts of sounding out words do not respond well to reading instruction, regardless of how it is presented.

Auditory dyslexics usually must begin with concrete letter forms, matching them, arranging them in prescribed sequences, and spelling out simple words the teacher provides as models. Gradually, by using tangible forms as the tactile base, pupils begin to associate specific concepts with the symbols they can touch, feel, and manipulate. Many teachers have clinched such learning by adding taste and smell with cookies shaped like alphabet letters. The point is that whatever sensory stimuli are necessary to imprint the concepts within the child's perception should be used.

Two effective decoding systems have recently become available to classroom teachers, and each system is highly successful in unlocking phonetic analysis (auditory memory) for dyslexics. *DISTAR*, published by Science Research Associates (SRA), combines several sensory input channels at once to give the student a multi-sensory foundation for identifying, then applying speech sounds to reading. Occasionally we see a dyslexic child who is confused by the *DISTAR* method, but this is usually due to inexperienced teaching rather than to the program itself. *DISTAR* has made reading a reality for thousands of disabled learners who had no hope of learning to read in traditional methods and materials.

Glass Analysis, developed by Gerald G. and Esther W. Glass, is published by Easier to Learn, Incorporated, Garden City, New York, 11530. This visual/oral approach provides a highly structured framework that teaches dyslexics how to identify important clues within word forms. *Glass Analysis* is often successful when *DISTAR* is not in opening the door to reading for handicapped learners. Each program is effective with adults and both are widely used in Adult Basic Education instruction.

Principle 3: Provide for Kinesthetic Reactions

Many teachers control their classes by the dictum "I want silence and plenty of it!" This mode of instruction is supported by those administrators who judge the quality of teaching by the degree of silence in the classrooms. Unfortunately, a habitually quiet class is actually a poor learning environment for auditory dyslexics. Certainly the noise level must be controlled, but, when body movement and vocal response are sharply curtailed, dyslexics are immobilized, so far as learning channels are concerned.

Several years ago Frank Riessman suggested a classification system for identifying behavior patterns found in every classroom.[1] According to his system, three different "styles of learning" can be identified. Number One is the silent learner, characterized by a mostly passive, quiet, unobtrusive manner that would have delighted professional librarians a generation ago. Number One learners gain knowledge (crystallize concepts) mostly through vision. They learn very well the silent way. During study time they want to be left alone. Number One's are seldom dyslexic, although occasionally we see disabled learners who fit this learning style.

Alongside the quiet students are the noisy minority, the Number Two's. These students must combine three learning channels simultaneously to crystallize concepts. They must see it, say it, and hear it all at once. If the noisy student is denied speech and hearing during study time, he does not completely internalize what he reads. He can be forced into submission by overbearing adults, but he will always subvocalize while reading, which is an active substitution for saying it to himself. The noisy students usually drive the quiet ones up the wall unless the teacher takes steps to separate them during study time.

The remaining small minority are the body learners who cannot cope with learning unless body motion and muscle reactions are involved. These learners must see it, say it, hear it, and manipulate or touch it before concepts crystallize. When forced to sit still and be quiet, they cannot learn. These students usually become discipline problems in traditional classrooms and are usually regarded as "hyperactive."

Auditory dyslexics are especially crippled when body involvement is denied in learning situations. A remedial routine developed by Lydia A. Duggins is highly successful in awakening perceptual awareness of phonetic values in dyslexic children. The entire body is involved as the child bends, stoops, whirls, jumps, skips, or crawls, making his body act out the sound-symbol relationships he does not perceive through passive hearing alone. Dr. Duggins' book, *Developing Children's Perceptual Skills in Reading,*[2] suggests a five-step routine for teaching short vowel

---

[1] Frank Riessman, "Styles of Learning," *NEA Journal,* vol. 55 (March 1966), 15–17.

[2] Lydia A. Duggins, *Developing Children's Perceptual Skills in Reading* (Wilton, Connecticut: Mediax Inc.), 1968.

sounds. The child stands *at* his chair for short a. He crawls *under* his chair for short u. He stands *on* the chair for short o. He sits on the *edge* for short e. And he sits fully *in* the chair for short i. As many clinicians have discovered, this kind of kinesthetic involvement is somewhat noisy, but it works. When the child's body moves in response to abstractions, he begins to understand what the phonics teacher is talking about. If an auditory dyslexic is forbidden to use his overall body as a learning channel, being forced to sit passively and "think," he cannot interact with the teacher's instructions. Rather than being a hallmark of good teaching, quietness is synonymous with illiteracy, in the case of most dyslexics.

Principle 4: Build a Stock of Mnemonic Cues

Even when they master the fundamental sound-symbol associations for decoding, auditory dyslexics usually do not become fluent spellers. This is because of their inability to retain clear visual images of word configurations. Because he does not "see" word forms when working from memory alone, the dyslexic has no reliable memory cue system for accurate recall of word configurations. In other words, when there is no visual model for him to see, the auditory dyslexic is helpless to reconstruct accurate word forms on paper.

Adult dyslexics who have achieved academic success have done so by devising their own systems for recalling specific spelling patterns. Few dyslexics ever tell about their private devices for fear of being thought silly. It does sound strange to listen to a dyslexic subvocalize while working out spelling patterns: "Let's see . . . 'mother' is t–h–e with *mo* in front and *r* on the end . . . . 'warm' is a–r–m with *w* in front . . . . 'there' is h–e–r–e with *t* in front . . . ." Because he cannot conceptualize sound patterns in printed symbol form, the auditory dyslexic remembers bits and pieces of spelling patterns, tacking on letters or clusters of letters to flesh out the skeletal structures he does recall.

When classroom teachers are aware of this perceptual peculiarity, they can help dyslexic children a great deal in the classroom. After assigning the week's spelling words, the teacher can help the children devise whatever meaningful memory (mnemonic) cues they can handle. It is completely irrelevant whether a pupil's mnemonic devices please or make sense to the teacher. The important thing is whether they help the child. If the pupil *needs* mnemonic aids, then anything else is nice or irrelevant and should be disregarded in the interest of achieving literacy.

Principle 5: Emphasize Consistent Spelling Patterns

An old-fashioned technique that is regaining acceptance is to drill "word families," which introduces children to stable, similar configurations that stay within the rules. Many teachers have used this technique under the guise of "consonant substitution" in basal reader instruction. The device is to present a root spelling form, such as the "at family." Then the pupils practice building familiar words by placing different consonants in front of *–at:* cat   bat   hat   rat. Many teachers shy away from nonsense words (lat, wat, or dat). Children, however, are usually delighted with nonsense word forms. In fact, most youngsters spend a great deal of their private fantasy time devising word games. In a form of solitaire, they mimic words they hear, creating nonsense vocabularies just for the fun of it. Successful clinicians have found making nonsense words a highly motivating activity for reluctant readers and spellers.

Even adolescents respond well to this activity, so long as the teacher turns a deaf ear to the *double entendre* items which inevitably occur. If things become too earthy with worldly-wise adolescents, the teacher should effectively stop the double talk at once. This is done by informing the culprits in a stern tone of voice, "I know *exactly* what that means, and I don't want to hear it again." Before calling a student's bluff, however, the teacher must be sure the student is consciously trying to be cute. Some naive youngsters (as well as teachers) have no inkling that their terms carry double meanings.

The important point is not to confront the dyslexic child with variable word forms that violate the rule of generalization he is trying to comprehend. For example, if he is coming to grips with the fact that when *o* comes by itself inside a short word, it has the sound of *o* in "hot," then he should not suddenly be exposed to the word *cold.* It is totally irrelevant at this point that "*o* before *ld* has its long name." This kind of generalization has absolutely no meaning to most dyslexics. Their mastery of sound-symbol relationships is built upon visual cues, not upon abstractions. In fact, even intelligent adult dyslexics usually do not become conversant with phonic generalizations. Teachers of dyslexics must realize that these unique students seldom respond to abstractions. Instead, learning procedures must be structured around a system of mnemonic and visual cues. If the classroom can provide for this unorthodox learning style, much can be done to help auditory dyslexics compensate for their perceptual deficiencies.

Principle 6: Provide Visual Cues

A firmly entrenched attitude among teachers is that tests must be taken strictly from memory, if we are to determine just what the student has "learned." Consequently, all visual cues to answers are removed, forcing students to retrieve information or synthesize responses from memory alone. This rather curious custom is unfortunately divisive, arbitrarily labeling talented test takers as "good students" and those who perform awkwardly on tests as "poor students." Those youngsters who are gifted with quick, accurate memory (retrieval) are the star performers, regardless of whether they can make practical application of their knowledge. In fact, the term "test wise" is often heard among educators, denoting the students who know how to pass tests, even when they do not understand the content of the questions. Also in current use is the cynical student phrase "multiple guess," referring to the so-called objective tests which force students to select one of several arbitrary choices.

Forcing a dyslexic child to work from memory alone, when his memory (retrieval) is erratic, is certainly questionable educational practice. When such a pupil can function well if given visual models for points of reference, then it is imperative that teachers provide this kind of reinforcement.

It is not really cheating on a spelling test, for example, when a dyslexic glances at the cursive writing chart to remind himself of how to make a certain letter form. This is survival. Neither is it showing favoritism for the teacher to display model spelling patterns while the class is doing written test items. If navigators must have trustworthy directional instruments to point the way to specific destinations, dyslexics must have visual cues. The purpose of education is to produce independently literate individuals who know how to read the signs and do what they say. Dyslexics are placed in hopeless situations when teachers hide all the visual indicators, forcing the students to work from memory. The same teachers would be horrified to see a track coach confiscate the crutches of a physically disabled child, and then force him to hobble after his able-bodied peers just to "test" his track skills.

Visual cues can be in the form of pictures, graphs, charts, colors, or textures—whatever is appropriate in the classroom situation. Regardless of the code, auditory dyslexics prove remarkably knowledgeable when allowed to work within reference distance of consistent visual cue systems. Without such reinforcement, they become understandably restless, uncooperative, and eventually hostile toward school.

Principle 7: Allow Oral Answers to Test Questions

Every teacher who reads this book can recall a personal experience of frustration in taking an examination. College professors are aware of the near panic felt by many adult students, including classroom teach-

ers, when forced to work strictly from memory in answering comprehensive test items. Physicians who practice near universities know when
qualifying exams are scheduled for doctoral candidates. Medical clinics
are beseiged by graduate students seeking relief from hypertension,
ulcers, and near collapse under the strain of taking tests without benefit
of visual cues. It is unfortunate that adults who experience such trauma
seem to have so little understanding of the feelings and needs of children.

Dyslexics in particular present the behaviors of worried adults at
test time. When required to write down or otherwise encode what they
should have learned, working entirely from memory, these students face
a difficult choice: that is, either to endure the pain and embarrassment of
flunking another test, or to avoid the test if possible. This intense frustration causes much of the ugly classroom behavior seen in dyslexics who
decide to fight the system. This sort of confrontation is not necessary.

When alternative ways to respond to tests are provided, dyslexics
usually exhibit satisfactory knowledge. Through listening and even reading, perceptually impaired students gain a great deal of accurate information. Classroom teachers who understand the dyslexic dilemma have
discovered that handicapped students can be held responsible for specific
information if allowances are made for their difficulties in reporting or
encoding. Oral tests have proved the answer in many classrooms. When
allowed to verbalize orally, without being penalized for dyslexic handicaps on paper, these students experience success, which, of course, is
what education is all about.

Classroom Activities for Auditory Dyslexia

Organizing the Classroom

Auditory dyslexics do not respond to the usual practice of presenting
a generalization, and then illustrating that rule through numerous experiences with symbols or words which follow the rule. Instead, dyslexics
must begin with structured experience. At a later time they may arrive
at the generalization, although many never are able to comprehend the
rules. They gain a level of functional performance without being able to
verbalize why or how they carry out certain language behaviors. Since
independent literacy is the goal of education, this functional level must
be considered sufficient.

All the senses must be involved in becoming a functional reader or
speller, if one is dyslexic. This immediately poses problems, so far as
classroom management is concerned. The teacher's dilemma is to pro-

vide for the different modes, or learning styles, she finds among her pupils. This can be accomplished if the teacher keeps her sense of humor, is not too rigid, and remembers that her pupils are human beings with exactly the same feelings she herself experienced in the toughest college course she ever took. If it had not been for mercies extended by sympathetic professors, many excellent classroom teachers would never have gained professional certification.

There are literally thousands of ideas in professional publications for teaching reading, writing, and spelling skills to perceptually handicapped children. The teacher of dyslexics must keep in mind the cardinal principles for these handicapped children: simplicity, repetition, and step-by-step progression into higher level skill areas. Almost any teaching technique can be made to fit the needs of dyslexics if the pace is kept slow enough and the drill work simple and thorough.

Before sound-symbol relationships begin to become functional with dyslexics, these children must experience myriad associations with stable word units utilizing the generalizations the teacher hopes to teach. The most manageable source of word units is the daily vocabulary of the children. It is a disturbing fact, yet one which educators cannot deny, that many dyslexics will never finish school. Therefore, they need to master the basic skills of functional literacy if they are to manage their own affairs whenever formal schooling is over.

Establishing a Utility Corner.   Basal readers, spelling manuals, language handbooks, and arithmetic and social studies textbooks are virtually meaningless to most dyslexic children. This is not to criticize the materials or their authors. The point is that texts designed for the average, middle-achieving student are not geared for the extremely slow reaction time of the dyslexic. Because of his different style of learning, the dyslexic's literacy skills must be geared to his immediate, tangible environment. Although he is capable of imagination, he is nearly always a physical learner (the body student) or an oral-aural learner (the noisy student), according to Dr. Riessman's categories. This being true, his quest for independent reading, spelling, writing, and arithmetic skills must take a different course. The most direct route is through the experiences he encounters every day, although this seeming detour away from textbooks traumatizes many leaders of established education.

The most effective classroom device for enlisting the interest and cooperation of auditory dyslexics is a utility corner, or whatever the teacher and pupils want to call it. This technique is as effective with adolescents and adults as it is with kindergartners. The need is to create a permanent place in the room where utility words are displayed. Two or three shelves of common grocery items are needed, displaying food labels which every citizen should know how to read and spell. Included are the prices, needed to teach simple computation. In addition to the grocery shelves are other utility items, such as clothing, utensils, tools, sports and recreation equipment, parts for motor bikes or cars, items for good grooming, common medical supplies, and whatever else is appropriate to the interests and life styles of the students involved.

In addition to these tangible objects, other utility word sources should be provided: sections of the daily newspaper; a Bible for religiously oriented students; mail order catalogs; phone and city directories; maps of city and state; travel guidebooks from major oil companies. For older students there should be ample checkbooks and budget planning materials; cookbooks; income tax forms; applications for fishing, hunting, and driver's licenses; manuals outlining local hunting, fishing, and motor vehicle regulations; and reproductions of traffic signs. There should be a browsing table for popular magazines the students bring to exchange, as well as comic books and paperbacks they have enjoyed. There should be a guide for television shows and reviews of movies, as well as current magazines on easy reading levels.

All of this is not for entertainment, and it need not occupy much space. The utility corner is absolutely practical, as well as essential for treating dyslexia in the classroom. The packages and other materials provide immediate visual cues through colors, shapes, word forms, and unique configurations. These cues trigger quick recall of important information for students with faulty retrieval. Here the teacher finds a wealth of simple, practical language materials for teaching literacy, which is the primary social need of dyslexics. Of course, it would be nice if the students could spend time with their textbooks. But until they can function in the marketplace, textbooks are largely irrelevant.

Even primary children need to master a basic reading, writing, and spelling vocabulary of utility terms. Perhaps every teacher should live as dyslexics live for a while, not knowing which door leads to the right restroom, not knowing how to find specific streets or house numbers, not being able to order a meal from a menu, not knowing how to deposit money in a bank or how to make or follow a shopping list, and not being able to write the simplest kind of letter. The utility corner opens up many new doors into face-saving independence, as well as providing the teacher with ready-made sources of instructional activities.

Every important phonics generalization can be taught from the utility corner. For example, the grocery shelves are loaded with word families: that is, the *–am* family (ham   jam   Pam   Spam   yam). Variant spelling patterns are easily illustrated: steak   cake   weight.

Homonyms are evident, particularly in traffic terminology: right–write wait–weight road–rode. Also at the teacher's fingertips are words to illustrate generalizations about dividing words into syllables:

1. Dividing between consonants that are alike (double consonants)
   but/ter   dol/lar   car/rot   ham/mer   pep/per   cab/bage
2. Dividing between consonants that are not alike
   tur/key   sil/ver   quar/ter   Hon/da   Mus/tang
3. Dividing after the vowel in open syllables
   ba/con   rhu/barb   pe/can   to/ma/to   Che/velle
4. Dividing between speaking vowel units
   Bu/ick   /Toy/o/ta   su/et   O/hi/o   ra/di/o
5. Compound words
   straw/berry   pine/apple   police/man
   ice cream   hot dog   post office

The utility corner is a prime source of creative writing ideas, if the quantity expected from dyslexics is kept small. With the many sensory cues from pictures, packages, colors, shapes, and flavors, there is a wealth of quick stimulus material. Dyslexic students find it much easier to write acceptably when this kind of cue library is at hand. It is personal because they have helped assemble the items in the utility corner. It is familiar because of the interaction and discussions triggered by the materials. The principal value is that this corner is theirs. It is not something the teacher has dictated from an impersonal, overwhelming text. With this sort of local authority on hand, the teacher is now prepared to hold her dyslexic students accountable for reasonable quotas of achievement, just as she holds other students accountable for material from their texts. In other words, now that materials have been accumulated to meet individual needs, it is time for everyone in the class to get to work.

Dyslexics should not be pampered any more than their peers. Once the teacher has provided learning sources within the skill ranges of her youngsters, dyslexic students can be held accountable for this material. If the other children are expected to master twenty spelling words each week from a regular grade-level text, then the utility corner students can meet a similar expectation, scaled down to their levels of literacy, of course. Occasionally the teacher will have a handicapped student who cannot cope with the same quantity of output as other dyslexics. His productive rate should be ascertained, and then he should be held accountable for what he can do at his own pace. Since some dyslexics work ten or fifteen times more slowly than others, productivity should be geared to ability to maintain a steady work rate.

The utility corner is only a starting place. If a student should not finish his formal education, at least he can shop for groceries or fill out a job application form. The hope is that by starting with a practical base in the utility corner, each dyslexic will eventually transfer his literacy skills to text materials. It is essential, however, that this transfer not be forced. As the foundations for literacy are laid, most dyslexics will want to move on to more sophisticated reading, writing, and spelling attainment. Peer influence is largely responsible for this kind of maturity. There is a reason why dyslexics in traditional classroom settings show so little interest in becoming involved in text and library reading. It is because such activities have been forced by anxious teachers before the students can handle these expectations with any comfort or pleasure. When a boy finds himself comprehending used car ads, or when a girl is able to understand a recipe from the back of a sugar package, then each is approaching the next step of independent reading, that of decoding comparable materials in book form. But this transition is extremely sensitive. When adults push too hard too soon for more mature reading behaviors, dyslexics revert to their old habits of avoidance and rebellion. The utility corner is largely a rest stop along the way. The purpose is to build self-confidence on a practical, day-to-day basis in the area in which these students really live. When they are comfortable, most of them will volunteer to leave the utility corner for less tangible areas of education.

Creating an Interaction Center.   Correcting auditory dyslexia in the classroom depends upon one vital element: interaction. If this factor is missing from the dyslexic's learning environment, then very little formal skill development will occur. Riessman's styles of learning suggest that several forms of interaction may be needed within a classroom. No one can expect a teacher, working alone with many children, to satisfy all the needs of her pupils. The utility corner is one way to stimulate certain learning styles into productivity. Establishing an interaction center is another.

Interaction involves physical movement, listening (auding), and speaking (oral-aural interchange). Auditory dyslexics must experience all three aspects of interaction in order to integrate the elements of reading, writing, and spelling. In other words, they need to feel it, hold it, manipulate it, hear it, say it, and act it out, if necessary. This cannot possibly occur at the reading circle or when the dyslexic child is confined to his seat.

The teacher's first problem with interaction is keeping the noise level under control. The quiet students, who learn better in silence, are greatly irritated and frustrated by movement and sounds elsewhere in the room. If the interaction center has some kind of acoustical control, the sounds of interchange can be tolerated within the classroom.

Hundreds of classroom teachers have discovered an inexpensive way to muffle sounds, at least partially. The result is both colorful and restful. At certain times of the year large furniture stores and interior decorating firms discard samples used to demonstrate various brands of carpeting. For little or no cost teachers can obtain these remnants and sample pieces, accumulating enough odd shapes and colors to carpet several square yards in a corner of the classroom. Putting the carpet mosaic together can be a class project. Adhesive tape, such as wide plumber's tape, can be used to stick the pieces together on the back side. When turned upright the carpet mosaic provides an oasis of muffled noise, allowing the body learners some "wiggle room" without creating an overall disturbance.

Whatever means the teacher uses to achieve moderate acoustical control, it is usually possible to create an interaction center within a regular classroom, if only for a few minutes at a time. Ideally, the center should be partially screened by bookshelves or portable screens. The point is to insulate the quiet learners from the active ones. If the teacher counsels the children about accepting each other's needs, this arrangement usually proves satisfactory. It will not be perfect, but few teachers are accustomed to perfect conditions anyway.

The interaction center is primarily for the purpose of oral and kinesthetic interchange. For ten or fifteen minutes each day the teacher meets those pupils who need body involvement for comprehension. This is the place to try Dr. Duggin's kinesthetic techniques for comprehending vowel qualities. This is also the place to let dyslexics use their body cues in role playing as they try to associate meaning with symbols: *hop* as you say each letter to learn h—o—p; *skip* four times to learn s—k—i—p; *roll over* four times to learn o—v—e—r. When children are involved in this kind of body learning, an amazing growth in literacy often occurs. Once the combined learning channels have imprinted the concept in the child's conscious mind, it is usually there to stay, except in cases of agnosia or aphasia (see Glossary). The interaction center can accomplish more in a month than a quiet, passive remedial reading class can produce in a year in most cases of auditory dyslexia.

A remarkable discovery has been made by a number of teachers who have provided interaction centers in their rooms. A sturdy rocking chair can become an avenue of learning, particularly for hyperactive children. Many dyslexics feel themselves becoming more and more tense as the school day wears on. In fact, these hypertensive youngsters talk in terms of feeling "like I'm about to explode." There is no provision made in most classrooms for releasing this pent-up energy without creating a disruptive situation which distracts other students. The rocking chair is an ideal lightning rod for discharging potentially destructive friction in handicapped learners. An agreement is usually made that, when no one else is using the rocker, a child who finds himself tense may take his book to the interaction center. There he may rock and read for a few minutes until he feels like returning to his seat. If the rocker is placed on carpeting there is almost no noise to disturb other children at work. In many classrooms the rocking chair has helped save the sanity of hypertensive children and harassed teachers. The by-products are increased learning, decreased disruptive behavior, and remarkably improved achievement levels of those who need to rock away inner frustrations of the moment.

A classroom provision like an interaction center creates a new possibility for both teacher and pupil. For the first time there are alternate behavior modes possible. This means that dyslexics who generate frictions when they rub their associates the wrong way because of skewed perception now have an alternate route for dispersal of their tension. Ordinarily the teacher either bottles up her irritations or immediately strikes out at the offending child. If she holds back her true feelings, genuine hostility develops toward the child. He in turn senses the teacher's attitudes beneath her efforts to be civil, and he naturally resents and fears her authority. Sooner or later their relationship disintegrates into a confrontation which not only causes further deterioration of their mutual feelings but also upsets other students and adults involved. This is the universal dilemma of how to coexist with disabled learners in the classroom. In a class environment where there are no alternatives, there is virtually no joy, and usually very little learning.

Although it is difficult to provide well-stocked utility corners and interaction centers within already crowded classrooms, the effort to do so pays generous dividends. Merely demonstrating to disabled students that their needs are being considered is sometimes enough to create a positive working relationship between students and teacher. The major problems of teaching and learning may persist, but efforts to provide alternatives almost always result in academic progress, even when the teacher cannot provide for all the needs she sees in her room. Remediation of dyslexia begins with removal of inner barriers within the attitudes and expectations of adults and children. The teacher need not be concerned so much with the facilities at hand, as with new outlets to drain off the frustrations of dyslexia in the classroom.

Making Sound-Symbol Associations

The point has been made that correction of auditory dyslexia requires a multisensory approach involving all the senses that can be brought into active participation in the learning process. The three most basic learning channels are sight, sound, and touch. When these sensory pathways are integrated, auditory dyslexics begin to comprehend what reading, spelling, and writing are all about. The *DISTAR* and *Glass Analysis* programs are excellent commercial products for this kind of remediation.

Identifying Sound Units in Spoken Words. Some teachers think only of consonants and vowels when reference is made to sound units in spoken words. These elements of language instruction are not the beginning points for auditory dyslexics. Instead, beginning emphasis must be placed upon hearing syllables, or whole word units. If sight, sound, and touch can be brought together in this experience, correction of tone deafness to word elements is possible in the classroom.

Hundreds of activities for teaching awareness of word elements to dyslexics can be found in professional literature, but the emphasis is the same. The child must integrate the visual configuration of a word unit with its oral-aural counterpart. This is most effectively done by incorporating muscle reactions through the hands, feet, mouth, or whole body. Even for dyslexic adults the process is the same: say it, hear it, somehow feel it, and if necessary act it out. At any rate, an integrated variety of sensory impressions must be poured into the learning activity.

Stepping Off the Syllables. For many years younger children have been drilled in word perception through games. These are often accompanied by music, as in simple kindergarten games in which body movements keep time with chanted lyrics. Skipping the rope while chanting a rhyme is a playground activity illustrating this principle. But, because there are no visual configurations of the words or syllables being reacted to, such games seldom lead dyslexic children to make sound-symbol associations.

Beginner pupils are frequently given corrective instruction when letters or words are placed on the floor. Then the children hop, skip, or jump from letter to letter (or word to word) while singing a song or chanting a rhyme. This simple activity is quite effective in imprinting alphabetic sequence or a basic sight-memory vocabulary into automatic memory responses. Variations of this technique are used in restoration therapy with victims of stroke, brain injury, or paralysis. Certain forms of aphasia are successfully treated through whole body responses of this nature. For older dyslexics who are extremely self-conscious, however, less obvious routines are needed in the classroom.

Tapping Out the Syllables.   Probably the most effective classroom technique for teaching children to identify discrete portions of words is arm tapping or chin bumping. First the printed word is displayed, along with pictures and brief explanations of its meaning. The pupils repeat the word as the teacher monitors to be sure everyone is perceiving the pronunciation correctly. Then, if the word is of two or more syllables, the group practices tapping out the syllables, keeping time with their own pronunciations. For some reason, clapping the hands is not always effective with dyslexics. Tapping, as described below, seems more universally effective than clapping.

For example, *turkey* would be broken into two sound units. Care would be taken not to cause a child to think in terms of two words. A picture would be displayed along with the word which is printed on a flash card. The teacher would separate the syllables visually by cutting the word, allowing the syllable units to be moved apart and back together. This would illustrate how the discrete units go together to form the whole word unit. Then the pupils would use the first two fingers of the writing hand to tap the opposite forearm (left-handed pupils would tap with their left hands). Sometimes a very light tap is enough. Occasionally a dyslexic child will react only to a sharp slapping of his fingers against his forearm. The important thing is that he get a simultaneous, three-part sensation: vision, sound, and touch.

It is important that the teacher move the syllable cards in time to the oral pronunciation of each syllable. The dyslexic children must see the syllables actually blending together to form the word at the same moment they feel their fingers tap their arms. All of this occurs with the vocal rhythm of saying the syllables. The teacher will be aware of how much of this drill each word requires. Simple words like *turkey* will require minimal drill. More complicated words like *unconscious* call for considerably more drill involving sight, sound, and movement.

Counting Chin Bumps.   An alternate activity is chin bumping, used many years ago to teach syllabication. Instead of tapping fingers against his forearm, the student says the word slowly, feeling the drop of his chin as he finishes saying each syllable. This often calls for exaggerated speech so the chin movement will be obvious. This simple technique of marking oral syllables is so reliable, in fact, that it can be used with surprising accuracy. In applying readability formulas to establish the difficulty levels of library materials, researchers often count their chin bumps rather than rely on visual syllable counts. The disadvantage is that chin bump syllables do not always match dictionary syllable division. Dictionary usage is based more upon traditional language rules than upon the oral qualities of word production. Chin bumping and arm tapping, however, are tried-and-true classroom techniques for integrating sight, sound, and body movements to overcome dyslexic handicaps in perceiving sound-symbol relationships.

An essential outcome of tapping or chin bumping is the ability to track through the sequence of sounds accurately. As described in Chapters 1 and 3, auditory dyslexics tend to garble the pronunciation of many common words. Involved in this deficiency is failure to follow the sequence of sound elements through spoken word units. Tapping out syllables provides excellent corrective training for faulty sequence. For example, if the child fails to detect middle syllables, he should tap or count his chin bumps while the teacher moves the syllable cards together. If he fails to identify a syllable accurately, the teacher does not move the visual cue card. Thus the child has a visual reminder of his oral-aural deficiency. He is also confronted by a structured, tangible guideline for correcting this perceptual error.

Some dyslexics must stay with this basic kind of perceptual practice for many months. Others quickly learn to transfer these recognition skills to whatever materials they encounter in reading. It is important that teachers *not* mix traditional phonics with syllable identification. It is essential that auditory dyslexics approach word analysis from the whole word (or whole syllable) angle first. Once they have comprehended how syllables go together to make up word units, then they can begin to break syllable units into individual vowel or consonant elements.

Using the Typewriter and Tape Recorder. The value of the typewriter in the elementary classroom has only recently been recognized by educators. Because of the cost of new machines, most teachers have simply put out of their minds the possibility of having a typewriter in the classroom. Traditional school emphasis upon penmanship for everyone has further obscured the potential that typewriters hold for remediation of dyslexia.

As discussed in Chapters 4 and 7, dysgraphic students are especially handicapped by their inability to cope with the handwriting expectations of most teachers. Auditory dyslexia poses a similar threat for those who cannot recall word patterns correctly. When disabled students are given the alternative for encoding through a machine, a new world of possibilities emerges.

As our culture approaches the twenty-first century, there is less and less need for mastery of traditional penmanship. Electronic firms that specialize in business machines are predicting the obsolescence of handwriting in the foreseeable future. With new families of electronic devices already in production, it is conceivable that dysgraphic and dyslexic persons will be able to enter professions that now require spelling, handwriting, and composition skills. In an era of voice recorders and automatic typing machines, which offer a variety of options for encoding messages and retrieving information, the elementary classroom should at least introduce children to alternative forms of encoding and decoding.

Every classroom needs at least one typewriter, along with a tape recorder equipped with earphones for privacy. This equipment need not be new or expensive. In fact, it is better to have an old typewriter that cannot be damaged easily. His extremely slow work rate will force the dyslexic child to "hunt and peck" when typing out words. The emphasis is never upon typing speed, but rather upon encoding letters in correct sequence to spell out words accurately.

Several commercial typing programs are already being marketed for elementary children. It is not necessary for the classroom teacher to purchase such materials, however, unless she intends to teach formal typing skills. The typewriter in the classroom is not intended to replace penmanship. Its value with dyslexics is in giving physical reinforcement of visual and auditory patterns in words. When integrated with a tape recorder, the typewriter can be a valuable adjunct to the utility corner and interaction center.

For only a few dollars a sturdy, older machine can be obtained for elementary use. Often high school business departments can arrange for a few old machines to be kept rather than traded in for new ones, as is usually done. Typewriter firms sometimes have machines ready to be discarded. So long as the keys work and the carriage moves, the machine would be suitable for remedial work with dyslexics. The typewriter should be set on sound-absorbing material so it will not distract other students in the room. A piece of foam plastic will absorb almost all the vibration and noise, leaving only a faint "thunking" sound when the keys are struck.

The typewriter-tape recorder routine is quite simple. The point of this activity is to provide an integrated experience with sight, sound, and touch. The words can be taken from any source, preferably from the student's own vocabulary needs. The routine is for the dyslexic to study a word on a card, pronouncing the word into the microphone of the tape recorder. Then he spells the word aloud into the recorder. He types it immediately, referring to the model card as often as he wishes. Next he reads into the microphone the way he has typed the word. He then selects another word card, and he repeats this process. After spelling out five words, he runs the tape back to the starting position and listens to his recorded performance. The student continues this routine, five words in each work segment, until he has done all the words in his card set.

Almost immediately dyslexics using the typewriter become aware of the sequence of letters within the words being typed and recorded. Any reversal or rotation tendencies will quickly become apparent. The teacher may overhear a student muttering as he hunts and pecks away behind his earphones: "Where's the b? Uh, oh! I got it upside down again. Now, where's o? a–b–o–v–e. Above!" This stream of chatter is almost exactly the thought patterns a dyslexic child experiences with every school assignment. Listening to an auditory dyslexic work his way through an exercise with the typewriter and recorder will reveal much about dyslexic confusion with symbols.

Recruiting Teacher Aides

The Old Testament records a remarkable lesson in how a frustrated, overworked leader solved a major problem of group management. Moses tried to handle all the details, giving personal attention to the needs of a million people. Jethro, observing his son-in-law struggling to do everything himself, gave his famous advice: Divide the people into groups, and then appoint aides to take care of their everyday needs. In essence, Moses was taught how to conserve his strength for the major decisions his subordinates could not make. Because the plan worked, Moses became one of the giant figures of world history.

Like Moses, classroom teachers face a multitude of responsibilities, problems, challenges, frustrations, and even failures. When dyslexia enters the picture, a teacher must accept help. Regardless of her enthusiasm and personal resolve, no teacher can possibly meet all the demands posed by the different learning styles in her room. Help must be found and accepted. It is not a sign of strength for harrassed teachers to reject assistance in meeting the needs of disabled learners. In fact, it is difficult to defend a situation which pits a lone adult against the myriad needs of a roomful of children.

Using Older Students. One of the strengths of one-room rural schools was the interaction between older students and primary pupils. My own experiences as a student in a one-room country school have served as a lifelong model for behavior management. Mrs. Kiethley could have worked herself into an early grave had she attempted to teach all her students in all eight grades in that one large room. However, she demonstrated the wisdom of delegating responsibility. It was a signal honor to be an upper classman in her school. When his deportment proved acceptable, an upper-grade student would frequently be called upon to "listen to little Johnny recite." This was a cue for the older student to take one of the little ones to the cloakroom, out to the shed, or in good weather down to the creek. There he would drill the younger pupil until the child was ready to recite for the teacher. It was old-fashioned, to be sure, but extremely effective in establishing accurate perceptual awareness of phonics, arithmetic, spelling patterns, history facts, or whatever needed to be mastered.

There was a double purpose in Mrs. Kiethley's classroom management, of course. She did not call upon only the better students to tutor. Quite often an adolescent boy, struggling with elementary reading or spelling skills, would be assigned the task of teaching the alphabet to a child in second grade. Or a fifteen-year-old might be called upon to teach multiplication facts to a nine-year-old. This pairing of tutor and learner was intended to reinforce the older student's skills, as well as to accelerate the younger pupil's achievement. In other words, Mrs. Kiethley was practicing an age-old principle: We learn much better the things we are required to teach to others.

Many schools are remembering these old techniques in today's struggle to solve the dilemma of dyslexia in the classroom. By using older students as tutors, many teachers are finding a way to provide one-to-one attention for disabled learners. There is tremendous motivation for a sixth-grade boy to be asked to visit a primary classroom three times a week to teach a child the alphabet. Upper-grade teachers are witnessing changed attitudes in older students who now feel needed and involved, many of them for the first time in their school experience. It is impossible to say who benefits more, the tutor or the child receiving this individual attention. Both students tend to grow in academic skills.

Teachers have generally backed away from this sort of pupil-to-pupil teaching relationship on the grounds that only experienced teachers are qualified to give instruction. Although this may be true, so far as new concepts and overall education are concerned, it is not always true that teachers are the best guides for discrete skill development. In fact, older dyslexics often prove more effective tutors and monitors than professional adults. One dyslexic can express abstract ideas in a vernacular that is readily comprehended by another child. Adults frequently find themselves unable to communicate so simply or so well.

An important two-way exchange occurs when an older student monitors practice work with a primary pupil. First, an essential ego boost is gained by the older child who has struggled so hard and achieved so little. Being selected as a student aide usually does a great deal to awaken self-confidence and interest in learning. Second, the younger child is usually delighted and somewhat awed to have a "big kid" all to himself as his very own tutor. This is particularly effective when the older child is good at sports, or has won some sort of public recognition.

The point is that harried teachers have a ready-made tutorial staff waiting to be recruited. Care must be taken, of course, not to use immature students who are not ready to handle a tutoring situation. If a personal clash develops, if there is lack of sufficient discipline, or if some other factor makes effective tutoring and learning impossible, then the relationship should be terminated immediately. Usually, however, enough capable older students can be enlisted to give every dyslexic in the class twenty or thirty minutes of individual help two or three times each week. As Moses was relieved to discover, his new aides took much of the backbreaking labor off his shoulders. Then he was able to devote himself to the larger problems affecting the entire group.

Enlisting Adult Volunteers. Increasingly in America, national attention is becoming focused upon service to mankind, as opposed to satisfying one's own desires exclusively. Consequently, thousands of adults of all ages are interested in donating a few hours each month to a worthy cause. In every community there are interested high school students, housewives, working men with time to spare, and retired professional people who often feel unneeded by society. Schools near college campuses have still another prime source of energetic young talent, including many prospective teachers. There is no need for a classroom teacher to pine away for lack of help, in most cases. Teaching aid is more readily available now than at any time in our history. Teachers and administrators who have taken the initiative to enlist tutorial volunteers have not been disappointed, as a rule. There is always some risk involved when outsiders are invited in. Professional teachers, however, usually do not find this to be a serious problem.

The main difficulties in enlisting volunteers are finding adequate space for one-to-one tutoring and having time to give the aides sufficient guidance regarding specific details of their work with the children.

Once these volunteers have settled into a regular tutoring experience, they need surprisingly little direct attention from the classroom teacher. They are monitoring basic drills, not teaching new concepts.

The most effective procedure is for the classroom teacher to work through a committee of interested mothers who have time for telephoning and other management details. Parents of dyslexic children are the most helpful volunteer aides, as a rule. It is almost never wise for a parent to work with his own child. It is a rare parent who can remain calm as his own flesh and blood struggles with symbol mastery. Emotions are too near the surface between dyslexic children and their nearest of kin. When this is taken into consideration, tutoring assignments can be made rather simply, so long as there is a relaxed relationship between adult and child.

Tutoring sessions need not take place at the school. In fact, it is often best for the child to leave the school premises on released time, working at a nearby church, at the tutor's home, in a library, or some other place away from curious onlookers. Regulations governing pupil absence from school must be strictly observed, and this responsibility must be understood by the volunteer aides. Once these basic problems of time and place are solved, however, the tutoring sessions usually continue with no disruption of the classroom learning atmosphere. Responsible volunteers simply appear at scheduled times and the children leave quietly. Later they return without attracting attention. When a smoothly functioning volunteer system is at work, the classroom teacher finds many occasions to feel thankful and relieved. At last her struggling pupils are receiving individual attention. And at last she can devote her efforts to concerns which usually go unattended when the teacher tries to do everything all by herself.

References for Further Reading

1. Ames, L. B. "Children with Perceptual Problems May Also Lag Developmentally." *Journal of Learning Disabilities* 2 (April 1969): 205-208.

2. Anthony, Jeanne, and Edgington, Ruth. "Classroom Performance Improved through Movement." *Academic Therapy Quarterly* 6 (Summer 1971): 423-428.

3. Arena, J. I., ed. *Building Spelling Skills in Dyslexic Children.* San Rafael, Calif.: Academic Therapy Publications, 1969.

4. Auerbach, Aaron G. "The Social Control of Learning Disabilities." *Journal of Learning Disabilities* 4 (August/September 1971): 369-378.

5. Banas, Norma, and Wills, I. H. "The Vulnerable Child Listens." *Academic Therapy Quarterly* 4 (Summer 1969): 311-312.

6. Bannatyne, Alex, *et al.* "One-to-One Process Analysis of Learning Disability Tutorial Sessions: Part I." *Journal of Learning Disabilities* 3 (September 1970): 448-456.

7. _____. "One-to-One Process Analysis of Learning Disability Tutorial Sessions: Part II." *Journal of Learning Disabilities* 3 (October 1970): 509-516.

8. _____. "One-to-One Process Analysis of Learning Disability Tutorial Sessions: Part III." *Journal of Learning Disabilities* 3 (November 1970): 576-585.

9. Bannatyne, Alex. "Why One-to-One Tutoring Solves Many Educational Problems in Traditional (and Other) Schools and School Districts." *Journal of Learning Disabilities* 8 (March 1975): 138-139.

10. Behrmann, Polly. *Activities for Developing Visual-Perception.* San Rafael, Calif.: Academic Therapy Publications, 1970.

11. Bryant, John E. "Parent-Child Relationships: Their Effect on Rehabilitation." *Journal of Learning Disabilities* 4 (June/July 1971): 325-329.

12. Bussell, Carol, *et al.* "Positive Reinforcers for Modification of Auditory Processing Skills in L.D. and E.M.R. Children." *Journal of Learning Disabilities* 8 (June/July 1975): 373 376.

13. Coe, Sister Mary Andrew. "Parental Involvement in Remedial-Reading Instruction." *Academic Therapy Quarterly* 6 (Summer 1971): 407-410.

14. Cratty, Bryant J. *Active Learning: Games to Enhance Academic Abilities.* Englewood Cliffs: Prentice-Hall, Inc., 1971.

15. Ehly, Stewart, and Stephen, C. Larsen. "Peer Tutoring in the Regular Classroom." *Academic Therapy Quarterly* 11 (Winter 1975-76): 205-208.

16. Ferinden, W. E., Jr., *et al.* "A Supplemental Instructional Program for Children with Learning Disabilities." *Journal of Learning Disabilities* 4 (April 1971): 193-203.

17. Goolsby, T. M., Jr., and Lasco, R. A. "Training Non-Readers in 'Listening Achievement'." *Journal of Learning Disabilities* 3 (September 1970): 467-470.

18. Heckelman, R. G. "A Neurological-Impress Method of Remedial-Reading Instruction." *Academic Therapy Quarterly* 4 (Summer 1969): 277-282.

19. Hurwitz, Irving, *et al.* "Nonmusical Effects of the Kodaly Music Curriculum in Primary Grade Children." *Journal of Learning Disabilities* 8 (March 1975): 167-174.

20. Kallan, Cynthia A. "Rhythm and Sequencing in an Intersensory Approach to Learning Disability." *Journal of Learning Disabilities* 5 (February 1972): 68-74.

21. Kass, C. C. "Relation of Early Language Development to Subsequent Reading Disorder." *Reading Forum. NINDS* Monograph no. 11, National Institute of Neurological Diseases and Stroke. Washington, D.C.: U.S. Department of Health, Education, and Welfare, 1971, pp. 65-70.

22. Kauffman, James M., *et al.* "A Resource Program for Teachers and Their Problem Students." *Academic Therapy Quarterly* 8 (Winter 1972-73): 191-198.

23. Kimmell, G. M. "Acquisition of the Auding Skills." *Meeting the Needs of Dyslexic Children, and Others.* Reprint Collection no. 2. San Rafael, Calif.: Academic Therapy Publications, 1969, pp. 29-30.

24. Kottler, Sylvia B. "The Identification and Remediation of Auditory Problems." *Academic Therapy Quarterly* 8 (Fall 1972): 73-86.

25. Lane, P. R. "Educational Therapy for Adolescent Nonreaders." *Academic Therapy Quarterly* 6 (Winter 1970-71): 155-159.

26. Laurita, Raymond E. "Rehearsal: A Technique for Improving Reading Comprehension." *Academic Therapy Quarterly* 8 (Fall 1972): 103-111.

27. McPhail, Gail. "Getting the Parents Involved." *Academic Therapy Quarterly* 7 (Spring 1972): 271-275.

28. Miller, M. Z. "Remediation by Neurological Impress." *Academic Therapy Quarterly* 4 (Summer 1969): 313-314.

29. Mitchell, Elizabeth. *Ideas for Teaching Inefficient Learners.* San Rafael, Calif.: Academic Therapy Publications, 1968.

30. Morsink, Catherine. "The Unreachable Child: A Teacher's Approach to Learning Disabilities." *Journal of Learning Disabilities* 4 (April 1971): 209-217.

31. Murphey, John F. "Learning by Listening: A Public School Approach to Learning Disabilities." *Academic Therapy Quarterly* 8 (Winter 1972-73): 167-190.

32. Neifert, J. T., and Gayton, W. F. "Prerequisite Skills for Use of a Multi-Sensory Method." *Academic Therapy Quarterly* 6 (Summer 1971): 381-383.

33. Parker, Therese B., *et al.* "Comparison of Verbal Performance of Normal and Learning Disabled Children as a Function of Input Organization." *Journal of Learning Disabilities* 8 (June/July 1975): 386-393.

34. Partoll, Shirely F. "Spelling Demonology Revisited." *Academic Therapy Quarterly* 11 (Spring 1976): 339-348.

35. Philage, Mary Lou, *et al.* "A New Family Approach to Therapy for the Learning Disabled Child." *Journal of Learning Disabilities* 8 (October 1975): 490-499.

36. Rawson, Margaret B. "Teaching Children with Language Disabilities in Small Groups." *Journal of Learning Disabilities* 4 (January 1971): 17-25.

37. Reichard, Cary, and Blackburn, Dennis. *Music Based Instruction for the Exceptional Child.* Denver: Love Publishing Company, 1973.

38. Richards, H. E., and Fowler, R. M. "Helping the Learning Disabled through Existing Community Services." *Journal of Learning Disabilities* 3 (November 1970): 563-569.

39. Robins, Ferris, and Robins, Jannet. "Educational Rhythmics: An Interdisciplinary Approach to Mental and Physical Disabilities." *Journal of Learning Disabilities* 5 (February 1972): 104-109.

40. Sapir, S. G. "Learning Disability and Deficit Centered Classroom Training." *Cognitive Studies: Deficits in Cognition.* Edited by Jerome Hellmuth. Vol. 2, pp. 324-337. New York: Brunner/Mazel Publishers, 1971.

41. Scagliotta, E. G. "A Special Organization of Learning for the Exceptional Child." *Academic Therapy Quarterly* 5 (Fall 1969): 5-10.

42. Slaughter, C. H. "Deficits in Cognition: Implications for Curriculum and Instruction." *Cognitive Studies: Deficits in Cognition.* Edited by Jerome Hellmuth. Vol. 2, pp. 90-108. New York: Brunner/Mazel Publishers, 1971.

43. Smith, C. B., *et al.* "Reading and the Home Environment—The Principal's Responsibility." *Treating Reading Difficulties.* Washington, D.C.: National Center for Educational Communication, 1970, pp. 4-12.

44. Worden, D. K., and Snyder, R. D. "Parental Tutoring in Childhood Dyslexia." *Journal of Learning Disabilities* 2 (September 1969): 482.

45. Wu, J. T. "A Multiple Group Setting for Ability-Grouped Reading." *Academic Therapy Quarterly* 6 (Summer 1971): 355-358.

46. Wunderlich, Ray C. "Resolute Guidance for the Learning-Disabled Child." *Academic Therapy Quarterly* 7 (Summer 1972): 393-399.

47. Zedler, E. Y. "Educational Programming for Pupils with Neurologically Based Learning Disorders." *Journal of Learning Disabilities* 3 (December 1970): 618-628.

48. Zweig, R. L. "Perception Training through the Reading Medium." *Reading Disability and Perception.* Newark, Delaware: International Reading Association, Proceedings of the 13th Annual Convention, vol. 13, part 3 (1969): 127-134.

chapter 7

Correcting Dysgraphia in the Classroom

IN SPITE OF RECENT PROPHECIES THAT A NEW DAY IS COMING WHEN handwriting will be obsolete, classroom teachers are very much concerned with a child's ability to communicate in written form. It may be true that today's primary pupils will function in an adult world where machines will do the encoding. Meanwhile, it is essential that children develop enough proficiency in handwriting skills to cope with the world of today. The ability to put one's thoughts into legible, articulate written form is still a live issue in the classroom.

As described in previous chapters, the dysgraphic child usually has an idea of what he wants to write down. He may even have a model from which he may copy. The disability is that he cannot manage to put an acceptable code on paper. His writing is flawed by broken letter forms. He cannot recall whether to move his pencil to the right or left. Instead of beginning at the top of a letter to make a down stroke, he starts at the bottom and marks upward. His circular motions go clockwise, which is backwards to standard form. In putting his thoughts into written code he tends to run letters together, telescoping until entire syllables are obscured or omitted altogether. At times he perseverates, repeating writing motions or letter forms until his work is nonsense. On occasion a dysgraphic student will be unable to make legible letter forms at all, filling the page with "bird scratches" which make sense only to him. Regardless of how hard the dysgraphic tries, he cannot satisfy the literate world because of his awkwardness in handling the handwritten code.

Correcting dysgraphia in the classroom is possible if certain principles of instruction are observed. The classroom teacher must keep in mind that dysgraphics are not just being messy or disrespectful. Unless the child has become bitter and hostile through repeated failure, he will tend to do his best each time he writes an assignment. The teacher holds the key to the child's attitudes and self-concept. If he does his best, but it is never good enough for the teacher, then serious damage will occur in exactly the same way damaged feelings occur when adults are forced to work for impatient, critical supervisors who are never pleased. If the classroom teacher can practice patience and long-range optimism, success can be realized over a period of time.

Principle 1: The Pupil Is Doing His Best

I learned a painful lesson about dysgraphia the second year I taught school. My sixth-grade students were asked to write stories built around "trigger words" written on the chalkboard. Wayne seemed especially interested in the project because the trigger words suggested a science fiction theme, his favorite fiction form. I graded the stories with my usual thoroughness, marking every spelling, grammar, punctuation, and penmanship error with fire engine red pencil. Wayne's story content was unusually good, but the mechanics were awful. At that time I had no notion of dysgraphia. My attitude was that every student could do good work if only he tried hard enough. I handed back the papers at the end of the school day, and then dismissed the class. As Wayne passed me I saw tears in his eyes. "I liked your story," I said. "Then why did you bleed to death all over it?" he sobbed, running from the room.

As a teacher I had failed to understand a vital fact: Wayne had done his best. The messy, smudged paper I had rejected was the best he could do at that time. In bleeding all over his surface mistakes I had failed to perceive that he had done his best for me, but that I had rejected him. His best was not good enough for my standards.

Like most proficient grown-ups, classroom teachers habitually regard their pupils as miniature adults. This frame of reference blinds us to many vital elements in educational growth. Because we assume that what we see is what really exists, our pupils are judged by the surface characteristics of neatness, punctuality, quietness, dignity, poise, and how well their work fits the mold. The stereotypes by which we judge student productivity can be cruel, if we mistakenly assume that imperfect papers are evidence that the child has not tried. Such rigid expectations may have some validity for children without disabilities. Sensitive students like Wayne, however, are hurt day after day, year after year, because their inability to fit the mold brings false judgment upon them.

The truth is they usually try harder than their peers who always make good grades.

How does a classroom teacher determine whether a child is doing his best? The only feasible way to make such a judgment is to note indicators of improvement. For example, if Wayne has always disregarded (failed to perceive) minimal cues in copying material, his work would be characterized by poor punctuation, failure to indent for paragraphs, disregard of capital letters, and misinterpretation of printer's cues (see Glossary). The teacher will know Wayne is doing his best when the child begins to perceive the minor details which affect comprehension. In other words, improvement must be judged by the small corrections Wayne begins to make on his own, after these deficiencies have been pointed out by the teacher. If over a period of time there are fewer and fewer mistakes with minimal cues, this is proof he is doing his best.

An essential factor in correcting dyslexia is mercy. Although mercy, patience, understanding, and forgiveness are not directly related to phonics or word analysis, these attitudes are of critical importance in the classroom treatment of dyslexia. The merciful teacher is one who begins to look for bits and pieces of improvement, instead of continuing to "bleed to death" over the multitude of errors. It is difficult for some adults to believe but, when Wayne begins to observe capital and lowercase letter forms, this represents a tremendous stride in achievement for him. What might be an inch forward for the teacher might represent a thousand feet of progress for the dysgraphic child. It is cruel and harmful to judge progress always by the larger increments. If a child must leap all the way from C to B to demonstrate that he is doing his best, there is no hope for the dyslexic in the classroom. When teachers can accept the small tokens of progress as being giant steps for the dyslexic, then mercy will begin to heal bitter attitudes, allowing additional progress to be made.

The first step toward correcting dysgraphia in the classroom is not more handwriting practice. The first step is for the teacher to believe that even the messiest, grubbiest papers represent the best the child can do under the circumstances. In other words, the teacher must forgive the child's deficiencies. Far too many adults hold active grudges against dysgraphic children, solely because their written work is messy. Once it is recognized that the student is actually doing his best, then it is time to work for improvement.

The secret is to scan the dysgraphic student's work for molecules of improvement: certain letters no longer reversed; punctuation marks now being used; capital forms where they are supposed to be. Many teachers have reversed their marking systems, using the child's favorite color to mark only his points of progress. A paper with no marks would signify no noticeable improvement. From this point of view, the dysgraphic would cherish the days when the teacher "bleeds to death" all over his work, heralding the fact that she can at last see improvement.

Principle 2: Handwriting Is Intensely Personal

It would be profitable if every classroom teacher could relive her most sensitive experience in which her writing was criticized. Adults, particularly teachers enrolled in graduate education courses, are extremely sensitive when their written efforts are being judged. Any professor who returns research papers, essay test responses, or written reports can testify to the acute pain experienced by adults who find critical notes on the margins of their work. It is not unusual for grown-ups to shed tears over criticisms professors have made. The point is that none of us is immune to feeling possessive toward what we have written. Editors are especially aware of the problems new writers face in learning how to accept editorial suggestions. Of all the sources of dread which professionals feel, having one's writing criticized, misunderstood, or belittled is among the most acute.

This universal sensitivity toward one's written work is reflected in the way adults carefully guard personal diaries and intimate letters. Although school work is by no means as personal as one's private notes, there is a common feeling of caution when people are required to commit themselves to written form. Oral communication is not remembered verbatim, and the speaker's clever use of intonation and mannerisms can distract listeners from any personal revelations that might be uttered. But thoughts put into written form become permanent. In writing, an intimate part of the writer's self becomes vulnerable once it is crystallized upon the page for all the world to see.

Sensitive teachers are aware of how this timidity in writing affects classroom behavior. From the earliest grades through graduate school insecure students slip up to the teacher to whisper: "Do you want to see what I wrote?" Teachers do great damage when they impatiently send these students back to their seats without glancing over the written material. Professors who do not take time to scan a nervous graduate student's first draft inflict similar pain. When students reach out this way, they are actually pleading: "Please don't be too critical. This is the best I can do. Is it good enough yet?"

As students achieve success, they need less reassurance from their teachers, as a rule. Repeated success with writing, particularly if one has rhetorical gifts, brings enormous satisfaction. Teachers always look forward to having students who write well with an interesting style. But this kind of success is not available for the dysgraphic child in most school settings. Since dyslexics are by nature hypersensitive, they often compensate by appearing indifferent to praise. In reality, they are hungry for the acceptance experienced by more able learners. When forced to commit themselves to written form, dyslexics have no defenses left. Writing becomes a threatening experience. If the classroom is geared to the high levels of penmanship usually espoused by elementary teachers, the weaknesses of disabled learners are fully exposed. Their choice is to muddle through, like Wayne, or to grow so defiant that they refuse to try. If they hand in their messy papers, the teacher "bleeds to death all over them." If they choose not to try, then they are publicly branded as lazy, careless, uncooperative, or even dumb. No matter which way they turn, they lose, according to their point of view.

The dysgraphic problem has been intensified by the educational stereotype of correct penmanship. In reality there can be no such thing as the "correct" way to hold one's pencil, or slant the paper, or sit in one's chair while writing. Neither can an adult logically dictate the angle at which another's letters must slant, nor the balance he should obtain between ascenders and descenders or circles and loops. The penmanship standards demanded by educators have been arbitrary, based more upon bias than upon perceptual reality.

In recent years one's handwriting has come to be recognized as a unique signature of his personality. Wayne slants his letters toward the left, not because he is "incorrect," but because of unique tendencies of his individuality. The size of the writer's script can have a definite correlation with his intellective capacity, just as the way he dots i's and crosses t's indicates specific character traits or dispositions of mood. It is remarkably presumptive for a classroom teacher to declare that a child is "wrong," just because his script does not flow like hers. A great deal of ignorance has been involved in handwriting methodology, particularly so far as dysgraphic children have been concerned. Fortunately, the term "correct" is being supplanted by the more realistic term "acceptable." Having one's best efforts accepted does not imply that further progress is not needed. But being labeled "acceptable" allows room for growth, a step at a time.

If writing is indeed a highly personal thing, then classroom teachers should handle the subject accordingly. The rule of thumb should be a pragmatic one:

> So long as the child's writing is legible, and so long as it is the best he can do under the circumstance, I shall accept it without

making him feel inferior. Gradually he will learn to write more acceptably in order to avoid embarrassment as he matures.

Principle 3: Respect the Student's Territory

A few years ago the world of anthropology was set on its ear by a dramatist who became a science writer, Robert Ardrey. In two fascinating books, *African Genesis* and *The Territorial Imperative,* Ardrey elaborated upon the research of Dr. S. V. E. Leakey, who spent his life tracing man's origins in Africa. Ardrey drew hundreds of illustrations from the animal world to support his thesis that man, like lower animals, possesses a strong territorial imperative which he will defend at all costs. Ardrey contended that this instinct to stake out one's territory, and then defend it against threatening intruders, explains man's behavior. According to this idea, every aspect of man's civilization— religion, education, politics, family, recreation, technology, and war—is governed by the territorial need. From his observations Ardrey inferred that, to be a wholesome individual, every person must have a certain degree of privacy (territory) in which he is safe from intrusion by outsiders. The theory holds that, when man is deprived of his territory, he becomes neurotic, ceasing to be a well-balanced person.

This idea has been explored by scientists like Konrad Lorenz, who raised various kinds of animals, observing and defining their territorial behavior. Studies like these have suggested some useful applications for education. There have been excellent learning results where territorial needs have been provided for in teaching situations. Regardless of one's opinions about the ultimate conclusions such writers draw, there is an immensely important lesson for teachers in the concept of territoriality in the classroom.

If teachers are to succeed in correcting learning problems in today's classrooms, close attention must be given to the interactions between frightened, insecure dyslexics and confident, somewhat overbearing adults. Few teachers realize that one adult alone with one child is often not a one-to-one relationship. If the adult is overbearing and the child is insecure, the relationship is more nearly five to one, explaining why some children do not respond to private work with some adults. When viewed through the perspective of territorial imperative, dyslexic behavior does indeed appear defensive because the disabled learner feels his territory (inner privacy) is threatened. This accounts for much of the disruptive behavior encountered by teachers of the perceptually impaired. Most adults do not hesitate to defend their rights (territories) against outside threats. Walkouts, strikes, professional holidays, and other forms of protest have become common among educators. If professional adults react in this fashion when their territories are violated, then certainly one would expect hypersensitive dyslexics to do the same.

The classroom incident with Wayne illustrates this principle. As his teacher, I had carefully "motivated" him to respond to the creative story assignment. I want to say that I coaxed him out of his shell. What actually happened was that he let me enter his private world of make-believe. I was proud of the expertise with which I manipulated the whole class into writing stories from the trigger words. After all, did they not decide to use my words instead of theirs? Until I saw Wayne's angry tears, it did not occur to me that I had made an unspoken contract with my students:

> If you will write a story as I've suggested, I'll read it carefully. I know it's hard for you to spell and punctuate accurately, but don't worry about that. The main thing is for you to express yourself—be creative! You can trust me to appreciate the part of yourself you put down on paper. I won't betray your trust!

Then I "bled to death all over it," as Wayne so well expressed the situation.

Because I was a young teacher was no excuse for my violation of this dyslexic child's trust. As a sensitive adult I certainly knew the pain and embarrassment of having my own writing (territory) violated by stern graduate professors. Not six months prior to that assignment I had driven home in tears of rage because a professor had belittled a paper I had written for his graduate course. The mistake I made with Wayne was not to respect his territory. I betrayed his trust by bleeding on his mistakes, and then I compounded the injury by saying, "I liked your story." He reacted as any wholesome person *should* react by thrusting me out of his inner territory. It was several weeks before he let me back in. There are times when classroom teachers never regain a comfortable relationship with students whose territories they have failed to respect.

If teachers are to gain entry into the inner space of dysgraphic children, they must establish ground rules which will govern the behavior of both parties. This is sometimes called a contract. Basically the teacher has a frank, private conversation with the dyslexic student, explaining the skills which need to be developed. She presents a checklist of the trouble spots in the student's work, along with samples of his work to illustrate these deficiencies. Then the teacher proposes alternatives, naming the kinds of activities available for correcting the problem, specifying the amount of individual attention she can give, explaining her grading system, and telling who the aides will be, if such help is available. At first not all students are mature or interested enough to receive all this information. The teacher must use her judgment to determine when enough has been discussed at one conference. The point is to present a simple outline of the child's needs, explain what can be done about it in the room, and specify his responsibilities in overcoming the problems.

There are myriad reasons why a student might be reluctant to admit the teacher into his confidence (territory). In the first place, he probably will not trust her to keep her part of the bargain. A wise teacher does not push to get in. There is nothing more devastating to a child who has trouble expressing himself than for an articulate, outgoing adult to bombard him with personal questions. The teacher should not try to pry answers from the student. If no interaction is forthcoming, she should take the initiative by making direct assignments on how, when, and where the corrective work will begin. As the child gradually digests the teacher's offer to help, it will dawn upon him that she is genuinely ready to accept him, weaknesses and all. At this point he will begin to open up in conversation. In fact, one of the dilemmas of tutoring dyslexics is how to persuade them to stop talking in order to accomplish drill work.

The gist of this principle is simple and direct. The teacher must not overwhelm the student, entering his territory before he is ready to accept her there. Until the child gives cues that he is ready for a more personal relationship, the teacher must confine her outward interests to simple drill routines, explaining whatever the student seems interested in knowing about himself. Above all, his written work must not be condemned, even when it is illegible. The teacher must devise tactful ways to require unacceptable work to be done again. This is best done by letting the student evaluate his own work against a visual model. Above all, the teacher must not bleed to death all over his papers.

When the classroom teacher genuinely respects territorial boundaries within her room, being careful not to betray the subtle trusts her pupils manifest in her, then great strides toward improvement are seen. Abrupt, impatient, and domineering teachers, however, see virtually no growth among the dyslexics in their charge. Such strong personalities usually do not realize the effect they have on sensitive children. Most domineering adults perceive themselves as excellent teachers because their rooms are quiet and their students busy. Such teachers should never be in charge of dyslexics. Territorial boundaries are so fragile in these children that a heavy-footed adult tramples down the fences many times each day without realizing the inward devastation her forceful ways are causing. In other words, teachers should be chosen for corrective work because of their skills in sensing the territorial boundaries of their students. Strong-willed adults should be placed with outgoing students who thrive upon competition for territorial dominance in the classroom.

Classroom Activities for Dysgraphia

Establishing Directionality

The primary disability underlying dysgraphia is the inability to comprehend directionality. This means that, when the child attempts to form written symbols on the page, he does not have a clear, automatic habit of proceeding from left to right, or from top to bottom. Instead, he tends to mark circular strokes clockwise, which is backwards from what educators call correct. He also tends to start at the bottom of the letter or numeral form, marking upward. Again, this is backwards to standard orientation.

There is nothing wrong with backwards orientation as such. If left alone to adapt to reading, writing, spelling, and arithmetic in their own way, most dysgraphic students would devise ways to cope with literacy requirements in our culture. The major obstacles around which they cannot move are the stereotyped expectations teachers hold regarding handwriting techniques. When these artificial penmanship restrictions are laid aside, the dysgraphic child becomes as able as most other students to handle himself as an educated person.

It is the school's hostility toward those who deviate from the norm that inflicts permanent damage in dyslexics. By the time a dysgraphic child reaches middle elementary levels his interest in developing writing skills has been extinguished, or he has become too defensive to respond to usual classroom procedures. The fight to preserve his territory (individuality) has absorbed all of his time and energy. There is little inclination in older dysgraphics to venture into the niceties of "correct" scholastic forms. Handwriting amenities have been perceived too long as the enemy responsible for the child's rejection by adults as well as peers. Dysgraphic children are among the most seriously damaged casualties of our educational system. Correction of their disabilities is a long-range undertaking, but it can be accomplished in most cases.

If a teacher wonders whether this description of the dysgraphic's plight is overly dramatic, she should listen as these children verbalize their feelings to clinicians. Visual and auditory dyslexics appear to enjoy school, compared with the feelings most dysgraphic pupils express. The difference seems to lie within attitudes of classroom teachers. Most youngsters can at least trace adequately or draw acceptable pictures, thus gaining a degree of respectability in the primary grades. But the dysgraphic child, who cannot coordinate his encoding processes, is without even these means of gaining acceptance. Not only does he have difficulty reading and spelling, but he also compounds his poor adjustment by being messy with his work. Correcting dysgraphia calls for a great deal of patience on the part of the teacher. Not only must she teach graphic skills, but she must also simultaneously convince the child that it is safe for him to try.

Mastering Handwriting Skills.   Regardless of the student's age or grade placement, there is an essential starting place to correct his faulty concept of directionality. He must begin with cursive writing. This proposition flies full in the face of elementary specialists who for forty years have preached that manuscript printing must come first. The reader should keep in mind that this proposal concerns the exceptional child, not the one who fits the mold of the majority. Since most children do prosper by learning manuscript printing first, there is no intention of upsetting their educational routine. But, if dysgraphia is to be corrected, cursive writing style is essential, regardless of whether the learner is five or fifty years of age.

For seriously dysgraphic children, those who cannot trace over a model without getting off the lines, a template for tactile training is required. This is a device which forces the child's hand through prescribed movement patterns to teach him to write correctly. A number of template kits are on the market, ranging from inexpensive cardboard items to metal sets costing several hundred dollars. The classroom teacher need not spend money for expensive templates. Some simple homemade teaching aids can be constructed for little if any cost.

Clay Tray—A useful, temporary template can be made by spreading modeling clay in a pizza pan or on a cookie sheet. If a more permanent model is desired, the clay can be dried in a slow oven or allowed to sit in the sun for several days. With a stylus (an orange stick or discarded ballpoint pen) the teacher traces the cursive alphabet lowercase letter forms in fresh clay. Then the dysgraphic child follows the teacher's pattern as she guides his hand. Over a period of time the pupil will form a memory pattern for writing these letter forms correctly. By offering tactile resistance the clay impresses upon the child's senses a visual image of how to turn his hand, how to double back on circular forms, and how to make the transition from one letter to the next. This simple template is within the budget of any classroom. If the tray is covered after each use, fresh clay will remain pliable and usable for several months.

Salt or Sand Tray—Another kind of temporary template can be made by covering the bottom of a box or pan with salt or sand. As with the clay, the teacher traces cursive letter forms for the child to follow. For especially dysgraphic children it is sometimes necessary to use gravel which gives a stronger tactile sensation upon the child's fingertips. Many teachers dislike this kind of teaching device because it is easily spilled. If the pupils are mature enough to use it carefully, however, it can fill a temporary need for tactile reinforcement of handwriting skills.

Wood or Plastic Model—Of more lasting value is a template made from a strip of wood or plastic. First the teacher writes the entire alphabetic sequence, as if it were one long word, with all letters connected. Only lowercase cursive letters are used at first. The letters should be large enough to allow easy movement of the child's larger writing muscles. A woodburning set is then used to etch the letter forms into the wood or plastic. This provides a groove to guide the pupil as he practices tracing the letter forms. The groove should be just deep enough to guide the child's pencil point or stylus. The teacher needs to incorporate stop signals at every point where the hand changes direction in writing the alphabetic sequence. Stops can be indicated by small nails driven into the groove. Blobs of wax or spots of bright color are sometimes used. Or the teacher might press small pits into the wood, causing the child's pencil to bump into the hole whenever he needs to stop. The point is for a visual-tactile signal to catch the dysgraphic's attention, telling him that he must change direction as he finishes the letter form. Artistic teachers often add colored arrows to show the new direction after each stop. Daily practice tracing over cursive models soon yields results as the dysgraphic child begins to comprehend directionality in penmanship. If the pupil can spend fifteen minutes each day tracing the entire alphabetic sequence, the teacher will begin to see improved handwriting rather shortly.

It is important that tracing time not deteriorate into busy work. The child must be alert to what the exercise is supposed to accomplish. Since most dysgraphics are physical and oral-aural learners, it is essential to integrate sight, sound, and touch into this corrective activity. As he traces the template model, the pupil must say each letter name slowly— not the *sound* of the letter but its *name*. This drawled out vocalizing can be irritating to silent learners. If it is impossible to isolate the child with the template, he must be taught to whisper as he traces: "Ayeeeee . . . Beeeeeee . . . Ceeeeeee . . . ." This old-fashioned drill may seem out of place in modern classrooms, but it has a special purpose: to teach the dysgraphic child directionality. If the teacher can keep this purpose in mind, she will feel less uncomfortable when this unorthodox training begins in her room.

Ideally the dysgraphic student should work with a compatible monitor, at least part of the time. As the student traces the template, the monitor should stop him occasionally to ask: "What letter comes before d? What comes after w?" By tracing the cursive pattern, verbalizing the letter names, and constantly observing the relationships between specific letter forms, dysgraphic children gradually develop a functional awareness of directionality, placement, and formation of letters. This is the foundation of literacy, as the school curriculum is structured today. This kind of primitive drill is the most direct way to establish handwriting proficiency in dysgraphic children.

Handwriting Models on Paper—Use of clay trays or grooved templates should be a temporary activity, continued only so long as the student is unable to write legibly freehand. After a few days of drill with templates, the dysgraphic child should begin tracing over a model of cursive style on lined paper. The teacher should make a handwritten cursive alphabet model on lined paper, with all letters connected, just as she did on the wood template. Many dysgraphics are insecure. Even when they have proved their competency in one kind of activity, they may be reluctant to transfer to a more advanced version of the same exercise. Tracing over the teacher's model on paper may produce negative reactions in some students. If so, the teacher must be patient as she helps them try the new activities. With her hand over the student's, she should carefully guide the reluctant child's tracing on paper.

Gradually most dysgraphics trust their new ability to work without the physical structure of clay or a grooved template. The teacher must not make an issue of taking away the first devices, even when she is sure they are no longer needed for accurate work. When dysgraphics are forced on to higher level skill activities, they tend to revert to the old fears of violated territory. If new corrective exercises take on the negative tone of pressure which the child associates with traditional work in which he has failed, the teacher will have lost her advantage.

The ultimate goal of this simple, rote drill with cursive style is to enable the student to write clearly without a model. This transition is made gradually, first by moving to a tracing exercise on lined paper and then on to copying the teacher's script without first tracing over it. Dysgraphics usually must spend considerable time copying. This phase of skill development is very slow, as a rule. The very act of consciously commanding the writing muscles to perform against their natural inclination is extremely tiring. A writing exercise may seem simple and brief to an adult. For the dysgraphic child, however, writing two lines on his paper may be exhaustive work. Whenever fatigue or rebellion emerge, the activity should be changed.

It is difficult for adults to comprehend the total energy expenditure sustained by dysgraphic children during writing activities. The fatigue factor is similar to that of a flabby adult who jogs a mile or swims ten laps in a pool. When the disabled learner lays down his pencil after ten minutes of concentrated work, he is as ready to quit as the winded adult who still has two blocks to jog. When teachers understand the enormous energy drain experienced by dysgraphics during regular school tasks, it will be easier to respect the struggling child's territorial needs. When a dysgraphic student says "I'm tired. Let's quit," he is usually making a trustworthy statement which must be honored if the learning climate is to be preserved.

Models at Far Point—Gradually the teacher should lead the dysgraphic child into copying from across the room. Confusion with directionality will be evident in this kind of activity. As the child's eyes move from far point to near point, he must maintain an accurate visual image of the configuration he is copying. This is a frustrating task for most dysgraphics. The main purpose of this kind of drill is to prepare the child to be able to do acceptable class work as he advances through the grades. Students are at a serious disadvantage when they cannot cope with copying assignments, particularly at junior and senior high school levels where there are numerous visual aids in science and social studies. Students who cannot take accurate notes from distant sources are seriously handicapped.

Problems with Eyesight—Dysgraphic students often have massive problems with vision control, as discussed in Chapter 8. Certain characteristics of letter formation, irregular spacing, ragged left margins, telescoping, loss of place, and difficulty with figure/ground control often signal problems with eyesight. I have seen dramatic disappearance of dysgraphic symptoms in numerous young people whose faulty vision was corrected for school work. Students who cannot control binocular visual movements, or who cannot maintain clear focus in sustained work (see Chapter 8), are handicapped in copying, workbook assignments, and writing activities. The teacher must make sure her students can see well enough to do written work before assuming that learning disability (dysgraphia) is the cause for poor penmanship.

Practice with Dictation—The ultimate goal, of course, is for the dysgraphic child to write clearly and with reasonable accuracy when taking dictation or when writing from memory (auditory-to-motor). This ability cannot be developed in one school term by one teacher, except in some cases at an upper-grade level. The weekly spelling words represent an ideal channel for emphasizing independent writing skills. When working with dysgraphics the teacher must let them know what they will be expected to encode. This means that elementary teachers should begin assigning one or two brief sentences which will be dictated at a specified time. It is important that this effort *not* be graded. This is a training procedure, the purpose being to enable the dysgraphic child to cope with higher level dictation which will affect his grades as he matures. During the year the teacher should expand the quantity of dictated material until the student is able to cope with five or six full sentences at one sitting. This kind of structured drill will definitely increase the dysgraphic's confidence in writing from memory without structured guidelines or models for cues.

Checking for Mistakes. An essential survival skill for dysgraphic students is knowing how to edit their own written work for errors. This is an especially sensitive area of corrective teaching because dyslexics often react strongly against what they perceive to be criticism. The teacher must provide ample opportunities to allow the handicapped student to check his own work against whatever model is being used. It is particularly helpful for him to check any work for which he will be given a grade. Spelling tests, arithmetic assignments, social studies exercises, or science quizzes are suitable for this purpose. If the dysgraphic child is taught how to use answer keys or other scoring devices, he will be able to protect his territory by being the first to see his failures. Once he has checked his mistakes, he does not mind so much for the teacher or other students to see his work. The damage occurs when the apprehensive child turns in work which he suspects is not perfect. Suspense builds up to painful peaks before the paper is returned. If indeed it has not been good work, his ego is torn once again by the "blood" all over his paper. Checking his own work first is a face-saving device which is very important to insecure learners.

There is no greater risk of cheating among dyslexics than among honor students. In fact, cheating is almost always a direct measure of the pressure a student is under to be accepted by the system. If the teacher discovers dishonesty as a student checks his own work, she should reexamine her values, so far as the importance of grades is concerned.

The presence of cheating is usually a reliable cue that too much emphasis has been placed upon achieving good grades. Insecure students resort to cheating in order to find acceptance within a learning situation. If the pressure is coming from the child's home, the teacher's options are limited. Aside from counseling the child, there may be little she can do to relieve his anxieties about grades. If the pressure is from within the school, then grade standards must be adjusted for the sake of the child. There is great value in having a dysgraphic student monitor his own work for mistakes, both to preserve his territory against outside criticism, and to demonstrate progress or lack of it. It is a regrettable educational loss when self-criticism must be denied because a student cannot be honest with himself because he feels rejected by the system.

Increasing the Quantity of Finished Work

Regardless of the classroom teacher's good intentions, no student can be fully protected. Sooner or later the dysgraphic must cope with arbitrary demands for finished work with no consideration given to whether he is capable of doing so. Eventually he must either cope with a heavy load of assignments or drop out of the system.

Raising Production Quotas.   It is not difficult for the classroom teacher to map out production schedules for dysgraphic children. This is best done on thermometer charts that resemble the large outdoor signs used to show how Community Chest campaigns are progressing. Movable colored strips are raised by degrees to indicate new classroom quotas the dysgraphic student is expected to reach. By using color codes along with other symbols, each child's production goals are constantly shown. Each week the teacher reevaluates her pupils' work. If dysgraphic youngsters are making sufficient growth, their quotas for the coming week are increased by a small amount. If a particular child has not yet conquered a specific dysgraphic problem, his quota remains unchanged. Occasionally the expectation must drop for a child who has become discouraged. The point is to cause learners to stretch in small increments to make sure that steady growth is maintained.

The key to growth lies with the teacher who must sense when her quotas are reasonable, or when she is expecting too much. If the child accepts the new goals in stride, all is well; he is ready to meet the higher output schedule. If symptoms of frustration and insecurity emerge, however, the new goals are still too high. The child's reaction to the thermometer chart is usually a trustworthy indicator of his readiness for higher productivity.

There need not be a great deal of bookkeeping or detail involved in maintaining production charts. If the child is working in three major areas—reading, writing, and arithmetic—then his production chart should have three thermometer columns, each equipped with a color strip that moves up or down to indicate changes in the teacher's expectations. Each column is labeled at the top by whatever subject the child is working in. Up the side of the chart are numerals with lines running across the face of the chart.

For example, if Wayne is expected to finish three written papers this week, the colored strip under writing would be raised to line number 3. If he is also expected to finish five papers for arithmetic, that strip is positioned at line number 5. If for reading he is to turn in four written assignments, that thermometer strip would rest on line number 4. Thus a clear visual monitor has been provided for Wayne as well as the teacher. On Wednesday she can safely ask how he is coming on his weekly work schedule. By comparing the number of finished papers in his folder with the color code on the chart, he has an instant check of how much more work he has to do before Friday afternoon.

Dysgraphic children can be held accountable for meeting their quotas because such a visual cue system is fair. The child knows on Monday exactly what the teacher expects from him that week. The teacher is relieved of trying to remember these details because her assignment is reflected on the chart. Her agreement with Wayne to honor his territory by not nagging him to do his work is able to stand. By reminding him each day to check his own progress, she is avoiding the danger of trespassing on his inner space, which occurs so commonly in the classroom. On the other hand, Wayne has no excuse for failing to meet his production schedule. This is a fair way to teach dysgraphics how to accept increasing amounts of responsibility. If they "goof off" during work time with their responsibility fully in view, they must suffer the consequences. As part of the working agreement the student already knows what the consequences will be. The teacher has already informed him of the penalty for failing to carry out his part of the contract.

This sort of visual contract is as effective in kindergarten as it is in high school. In fact, for many years industry has used similar systems of production reminders for assembly workers. Employees who receive incentive pay according to their output are far more productive than those who receive only a base wage. Teachers who work on a contract basis, giving worthwhile rewards for acceptable work as well as significant penalties for work failure, have been amazed at the differences they see in student attitudes.

It is hard work to nag students into doing their tasks. The clever teacher utilizes incentive programs that do the nagging for her. In a way the production chart is harder for the child to ignore than the nagging voice of the teacher. There is something about the silent, persistent presence of a quota chart that spurs most youngsters on to fulfillment of their obligation. This sort of self-discipline is critical for the dyslexic. Lifelong lessons in timing and self-programming are instilled when a dysgraphic child is held accountable by a production chart. When Friday afternoon comes, there is no way he can whine out of the truth. If his week has been wasted, he must face judgment. If his week has been spent productively, he receives his reward.

The quota chart also allows the teacher to present alternatives. It is especially important for the dysgraphic student to be allowed a choice of written assignments from which he can make a selection to submit for evaluation. If he has done several more papers than the chart requires, he should be allowed to hand in the papers he considers best for the week. Thus both student and teacher are allowed to save face. When given this opportunity to decide his own fate, the dysgraphic child cannot blame his teacher for low marks on his work. In turn, the teacher is free to make whatever candid suggestions she feels are necessary. When the full decision has been the teacher's, both she and the child are placed on the defensive.

Probably the most important learning derived from a quota system is self-discipline. Of all students in our schools, dyslexics usually are the least self-controlled. Their entire perception of life is a scrambled blur of events, pressures, obligations, and information, much of which appears disorganized and incoherent to them. Without a highly structured system that keeps their lives ordered, dyslexics seldom achieve a sense of well-being. Those adults who have succeeded in spite of dyslexia have learned how to order their circumstances.

It would be tragic if dyslexics were taught only how to read, write, spell, and compute. Their primary social need is for self-control, which of course includes literacy. Production schedules are essential for children who are not able to comprehend chronological time lapse in proper perspective. If these young people are to manage family budgets, job responsibilities, and leisure activities well, they must be taught the ingredients of self-control over a period of several years. This is one of the major contributions the teacher makes in correcting dyslexia in the classroom.

References for Further Reading

1. Arena, J. I., ed. *Building Handwriting Skills in Dyslexic Children.* San Rafael, Calif.: Academic Therapy Publications, 1970.

2. Behrmann, Polly. *Activities for Developing Visual-Perception.* San Rafael, Calif.: Academic Therapy Publications, 1970.

3. Carter, J. L., and Miller, P. K. "Creative Art for Minimally Brain-Injured Children." *Academic Therapy Quarterly* 6 (Spring 1971): 245-252.

4. Croutch, Ben. "Handwriting and Correct Posture." *Academic Therapy Quarterly* 4 (Summer 1969): 283-284.

5. Early, Frances. "Developing Perceptual-Motor Skills: New Uses for the Old Template." *Academic Therapy Quarterly* 4 (Summer 1969): 295-297.

6. Early, G. H. "Developing Perceptual-Motor Skills: Overburdened Cognitive Processes." *Academic Therapy Quarterly* 5 (Fall 1969): 59-62.

7. Enstrom, E. A., and Enstrom, Doris C. "Practical Teaching Methods for Primary Handwriting Skills." *Academic Therapy Quarterly* 7 (Spring 1972): 285-292.

8. Footlik, S. W. "Perceptual-Motor Training and Cognitive Achievement: A Survey of the Literature." *Journal of Learning Disabilities* 3 (January 1970): 40-49.

9. Goldsmith, Carolyn. "Rhythm in Neurologically Handicapped Children as an Aid to Learning." *Meeting the Needs of Dyslexic Children and Others.* Reprint Collection no. 2. San Rafael, Calif.: Academic Therapy Publications, 1969, pp. 19-24.

10. Johnson, M. S. "Tracing and Kinesthetic Techniques." *The Disabled Reader: Education of the Dyslexic Child.* Edited by John Money, pp. 147-160. Baltimore: The Johns Hopkins Press, 1966.

11. McNees, Margaret C., *et al.* "Modifying Cluttered Handwriting." *Academic Therapy Quarterly* 7 (Spring 1972): 293-295.

12. Mattos, R. L. "Some Relevant Dimensions of Interval Recording." *Academic Therapy Quarterly* 6 (Spring 1971): 235-244.

13. Mitchell, Elizabeth. *Ideas for Teaching Inefficient Learners.* San Rafael, Calif.: Academic Therapy Publications, 1968.

14. Mullins, June, *et al.* "A Handwriting Model for Children with Learning Disabilities." *Journal of Learning Disabilities* 5 (May 1972): 306-311.

15. Revelle, D. M. "Aiding Children with Specific Language Disability." *Academic Therapy Quarterly* 6 (Summer 1971): 391-395.

16. Slocum, A. L. "Some Basic Motor Activities for the Neurologically Handicapped Child." *Meeting the Needs of Dyslexic Children, and Others.* Reprint Collection no. 2. San Rafael, Calif.: Academic Therapy Publications, 1969, pp. 15-18.

17. Solan, H. A., and Seiderman, A. S. "Case Report on a Grade One Child before and after Perceptual-Motor Training." *Journal of Learning Disabilities* 3 (December 1970): 635-639.

18. Trexler, L. K. "The Trampoline: A Training Device for Children with Perceptual-Motor Problems." *Academic Therapy Quarterly* 5 (Winter 1969-70): 145-147.

chapter 8

Distinguishing Dyslexia from Other Disabilities

MANY AUTHORITIES STRONGLY OPPOSE THE IDEA OF INVOLVING CLASS-room teachers in the diagnosis of learning disabilities. No one would deny the risk that inexperienced observers might label a child erroneous-ly. Labeling is a serious educational matter, requiring the utmost caution on the part of those who work with perceptually disabled children. In spite of the risks involved, there are unmistakable behavior patterns which characterize certain problems encountered by classroom teachers. These sets of behavior symptoms (behavior syndromes) are distinct enough to allow at least cursory screening for purposes of referral. This chapter is designed to give teachers a trustworthy basis for referring students who seem unable to function within the regular classroom.

Because of her daily contact with children, the classroom teacher can play a vital role in the correct diagnosis of certain kinds of learning disabilities. In referring children for diagnosis, it is important that teachers be able to furnish detailed examples of behavior in the class-room, on the playground, during lunch time, on school outings, or wherever else the child has been observed at length. Without an accurate, detailed summary of the pupil's school behavior, specialists are often stymied in making accurate diagnoses of problems related to learning.

The checklists of behavior symptoms given in this chapter enable the teacher to make professional statements regarding a child's behavior at school. Even when a problem is not diagnosed, the teacher will have a reliable basis for seeking outside help. If used with professional dis-cretion, this information can prove invaluable in obtaining help for chil-dren who might otherwise go undiagnosed for specific learning disabilities.

Distinguishing Dyslexia from Late Maturity

We who work with preschool, kindergarten, and primary pupils are deeply indebted to Arnold Gesell and Catherine Amatruda for their pioneer work in mapping developmental milestones in childhood. I have seen hundreds of late-maturing children mislabeled and assigned to the wrong learning environment because professionals did not distinguish between late physical maturity and perceptual disability. Gesell and Amatruda's *Developmental Diagnosis: The Evaluation and Management of Normal and Abnormal Neuropsychological Development in Infancy and Early Childhood* should be required reading for all teachers and diagnosticians.[1] It is very important that immaturity (lateness in reaching specific milestones) not be mistaken for perceptual disability. Late maturers can "outgrow" their learning problems with time and the right academic environment. Children with learning disability cannot. Thousands of parents have been mistakenly advised that "Johnny will outgrow his problems. Just be patient and leave the teaching to his teachers." By Johnny's eighth birthday it is clear that he is hopelessly floundering and becoming maladjusted toward school. By his ninth birthday his teachers are calling for help, only to discover that Johnny's lack of progress has been due to perceptual impairment of a permanent nature. Primary teachers often can distinguish late maturity patterns from true disability syndromes if careful observations are made. Gesell and Amatruda have paved the way.

One of the most trustworthy signals of readiness for school success is the child's tooth structure.[2] There appears to be approximately eighty-five percent correlation between the age at which a child's "reading teeth" (top front permanent teeth) emerge and the time he masters classroom skills in listening, writing, use of phonics in reading and spelling, and arithmetic. Several hundred primary teachers have found this physical milestone to be true. A physical enzyme structure is involved in dissolving the roots of baby teeth, causing them to loosen and drop out. This enzyme activity occurs about the time the child is ready to settle down to the listening (attending) and producing tasks of first grade. A girl who is developmentally on schedule should lose her first baby teeth by age six-and-one-half, usually during the fall of the first grade year. Most boys are six months later than girls in reaching this milestone in tooth development. As primary teachers know, far more boys have

---

[1] Knobloch and Pasamanick, editors, Gesell and Amatruda, *Developmental Diagnosis,* Third Edition (New York: Harper & Row, Publishers), 1974.

[2] Research findings of the staff of Jordan-Adams Learning Center, 1968-1976.

difficulty with beginning skills than girls. As a rule, boys do much better in school learning after they turn seven. Educators clearly need to review the common practice of starting all children to school according to birthdate.

Approximately eighty-five percent of the slow learners, late readers, and pupils placed in slow achieving groups show late tooth development. These children often lose no baby teeth until age seven. I see many children each year who still have their baby teeth at age eight. In my opinion, chronological age (birthdate) is one of the least reliable guidelines for placing children in educational programs. Tooth development in relation to a child's age is 85% reliable in identifying boys and girls who will probably have difficulty with curriculum tasks on schedule.

For the classroom teacher, late maturity is a critical problem. Immature pupils cannot cope with grade-level expectations. They cannot internalize the concepts presented in daily lessons. They cannot yet transfer and generalize concepts, nor do they build a memory continuum of yesterday's facts as the stepping stones for today's activities. In Piaget's terms, they cannot conserve form nor can they manage transformations and reversibility. They are quickly bored, constantly restless, and overwhelmed by the load of the school day. They are not, however, children with learning disabilities. Their little bodies are not ready for school. It is cruel for a child who is developmentally a five-year-old to be forced to carry work loads designed for seven-year-olds. Emotional problems, rebellion, unpopularity with peers, insecurity, and low self-esteem are generated when children are placed too soon in full academic expectations. We have unwittingly been inhumane to thousands of children who should have waited another year or two before being plunged into the fast-flowing academic stream.

Gesell and Amatruda have given simplified diagnostic guidelines for establishing readiness for school. Their work supports Piaget's assertions that certain stages of readiness must be reached before conceptualization can take place in children. It is not difficult for teachers to identify preoperational (concrete) learners, those who must manipulate physical objects or count their fingers to add or subtract. It is not hard to find six-year-olds who cannot draw geometric patterns of the average five-year-old, or seven-year-olds who cannot trace patterns expected at age six. Poor vision in immature children is easily observed (see Jordan Vision Screening Test, Appendix C). Before a child is labeled "learning disabled" or "dyslexic," his maturity levels must be defined.

A rule of thumb can serve as a cautionary guide in determining developmental maturity in children. If a child still reverses symbols, has short attention span, displays poor fine motor control in writing, and cannot grasp phonetic principles after his top front permanent teeth have emerged, he is probably learning disabled. Eighty-five percent of the dyslexic children we see follow this pattern. Many classroom teachers have found tooth development closely related to the time when children are ready for full school learning. Once tooth development signals general body readiness for sustained curriculum learning, the children who still have problems are usually perceptually impaired.

Distinguishing Dyslexia from Hyperkinesis

A controversial learning disability has come to public attention in recent years, creating vigorous differences of opinion between educators and medical authorities. No one has yet determined the cause, nor is there agreement about the management or cure. For want of a better name, the behavior problem is called hyperkinesis (see Glossary), hyperkinetic impulse disorder, hyperkinetic syndrome, hyperkinetic disease, Minimal Cerebral Dysfunction (MCD), and Minimal Brain Dysfunction (MBD). In cases involving actual brain damage the pattern is called Strauss syndrome. Regardless of the nomenclature, the behavior pattern is unmistakable. Any classroom teacher who has tried to cope with a hyperkinetic child will never forget that experience. Until the past decade there was little relief for this bewildering condition in children. In fact, because of similarities to aphasia, hyperkinesis is frequently classified as brain damage. Successful drug therapy is now available to help these children fit into normal society.

Many of the behavior symptoms of hyperkinesis resemble aphasia, as well as certain aspects of dyslexia. Still another behavior syndrome, loosely called "hyperactivity," is confused with hyperkinesis. Hyperactive is an ambiguous term, generally designating children who cannot sit still. Although hyperactivity is a disruptive factor in many classrooms, there is a great deal of difference between the two disorders. The hyperkinetic child is indeed hyperactive, which means he cannot sit still. But a hyperactive child is not always hyperkinetic. This is a very important point when medication is involved. Drugs that control hyperkinesis (stimulants) are absolutely the wrong medicine for hyperactivity. On the other hand, drug therapy that helps hyperactive children (tranquilizers) will send a hyperkinetic youngster up the wall. This critical difference must be clearly determined or the teacher may find some seriously upset children on her hands.

Medical science has not yet determined the exact nature of hyperkinetic impulse disorder, as the problem is usually called by physicians.

At times the disability behaves like an allergic state of nerve tissues, in the same sense that allergic sinus cavities become inflamed when exposed to pollens or dust. Sometimes hyperkinesis appears to be a state of underdeveloped nerve tissues. In this case it appears that the insulating sheath surrounding nerve fibers was not fully formed at birth. Consequently, the nervous system is hypersensitive, reacting to minute pressures normal systems never feel. Most hyperkinetics outgrow this condition by the time they reach seventeen, although some never do. Experimental therapy with vitamins and trace minerals has sometimes relieved hyperkinetic symptoms, indicating the problems may be caused by deficient diets in some children.

Whatever the cause, the problem usually responds to medication by Cylert, Dexedrine, or Ritalin (see Glossary). Because of dramatic changes seen in children who have responded well to medication, more and more physicians and educators are willing to place hyperkinetic children in drug therapy. Teachers who have witnessed a remarkable transformation in classroom behavior through medication advocate its use for truly hyperkinetic youngsters. Ritalin or Cylert can make the difference between bedlam and order. With this kind of relief available for hyperkinetics, teachers see little logic in the protests raised against medication in the classroom. Drugs like Ritalin and Cylert are not habit forming, the only side effects being occasional insomnia (trouble falling asleep at night), constipation, and reduced appetite. In a few cases there is a reduced white blood count. These are such unlikely effects that most physicians consider them negligible, if the medication is well supervised by doctors and teachers.

Poor Scholastic Achievement

The important problem of the hyperkinetic, so far as the classroom teacher is concerned, is chronic academic failure because of incomplete learning. Skills are only partly developed. Concepts are only partially understood. The result is that hyperkinetics are actually semiliterate persons until they have matured enough to respond to academic tutoring. On standardized reading achievement tests, the hyperkinetic will often score at or slightly above grade levels in vocabulary, word analysis, spelling, and even basic grammar. His comprehension is habitually lower than the other subtest areas. This is partly because of his twisted self-image. In spite of a miserable opinion of himself, he still believes himself to be even more clever than his teachers. Therefore he tends to second-guess rather than apply his intellect to solve problems. Few hyperkinetic students become good scholars, unless they receive medication which allows them to develop adequate study habits. Sometimes in their adult years these persons make up for their high school deficiencies through adult education. Most hyperkinetics do not, thereby losing the opportunity to develop the potential which was masked during their formative years by the unfortunate behavior syndrome which alienated them from learning.

Dyslogic Syndrome

Hyperkinetics seldom demonstrate common sense reasoning. While this is also true of some dyslexics, poor common sense reasoning is an earmark of hyperkinesis. For want of a better term, we speak of "dyslogic," the inability to employ logic (common sense) in making decisions.

It is not uncommon for the dyslogic pattern to be misidentified as paranoia or even schizophrenia in adolescents. Paranoids are unstable because they constantly suspect plots against themselves ("Everybody picks on me"). Paranoids are habitually on the defensive. Many dyslexics develop true paranoid tendencies in adolescence if they have been abused by adults who have not taken their cluttered thinking into account. When hyperkinetic children are not successfully treated and managed before adolescence, they tend to become truly paranoid in their teen years. But the dyslogic syndrome is different from paranoia.

Dyslogic students believe they are right. They are seldom aware of the fact that their decisions are based on only part of the total evidence available. The value of having common sense is that the person utilizes all available data in making decisions. When a student's perceptual processes make it impossible for all data to be integrated into a working whole, then he cannot use full facts and details in making decisions. Dyslogic youngsters habitually make snap decisions, impulsive judgments, and inaccurate conclusions, but they do so sincerely, believing themselves to be correct. When teachers and parents scold or argue to the contrary, dyslogic persons immediately leap to self-defense. Tempers are usually very short in dyslogic individuals. By nature they are active, impatient, impulsive, "now" people who have no understanding of delayed fulfillment. They want what they want when they want it. They do not perceive how frequently their decisions are skewed and out-of-line with the best interests of their associates.

The dyslogic pattern greatly affects comprehension in school work. Snap judgments on tests usually produce low scores, often followed by vigorous arguments with the teacher as to why the student should be given credit. Adult effort to show the student where his reasoning was incomplete does little good. The dyslogic student cannot see the forest for the trees, nor does he see all the trees. His life is filled with conflict as he constantly finds his decisions and judgments challenged. Reading comprehension is low because he does not build complete memory patterns from details encountered on the page. Many mistakes are made in math computation because he does not heed the signs. Attention span is short in listening to lectures, sermons, or class discussions. The dyslogic student is unaware that he is a spotty listener, retaining only bits and pieces of the whole presentation. His version of television shows and movies is often remarkably different from what his peers perceive. None of this difficulty with judgment or common sense is deliberate, as is the case with true paranoids.

The dyslogic person is usually an aggressive, basically happy individual who just can't wait for all the pieces to be assembled. He is constantly bewildered as his decisions and values are challenged on every hand, but he seldom broods or remains unhappy very long. He is always on the verge of loud verbal battles, especially with parents and siblings. Dating and courtship are precarious because few people with normal reasoning traits can tolerate the abrasive force of being closely involved with a dyslogic friend. Of all dysfunctions of learning, the dyslogic syndrome is one of the most difficult to modify successfully. Busy adults run out of patience. Classmates get tired of daily sessions interrupted by defensive, illogical arguments. The dyslogic student's unpopularity with the group causes him to form social bonds with other dyslogics.

It is virtually impossible to convince the dyslogic person that his judgment is faulty. If he could perceive this flaw in himself, he would not be dyslogic. This circular predicament makes rehabilitation very difficult. In working with a broad spectrum of convicted felons and delinquents, I have found the dyslogic syndrome in a large majority of inmates and persons on probation. It is impossible to convince a dyslogic offender that his poor common sense reasoning is to blame for his problems. Psychologists generally give up on these individuals who constitute the majority of our prison and delinquent populations. Teachers and counselors face a losing battle trying to argue with dyslogics who simply cannot believe that they are to blame.

The distinguishing characteristic between dyslogic problems and dyslexia is that most dyslogic students find their symbol processing capabilities intact. As a rule, they do not reverse symbols, scramble sequence, or manifest tone deafness to phonics. They are often avid readers and are usually quite intelligent. In fact, the dyslogics I see in private practice usually score within the superior range on intelligence tests. They invariably do quite well on brief, isolated test items. Their problem is that they cannot exercise long-term common sense to an effective degree. Their life goals are unrealistic. Dyslogic teen-agers seldom have a functional sense of money, how much it costs to keep up an apartment and a car, or how much is deducted from gross wages before net pay is in hand. They are dreamers regarding the future, fully believing their unrealistic expectations will come true. Many teen-age marriages result when dyslogic adolescents believe they can live in style on a gross income of $95.00 per week from a part-time job. They tend to use drugs and alcohol recklessly, believing that "this stuff can't hurt *me.*" They are seldom dependable on the job because their immediate wishes come before job loyalty. When their dreams do not materialize, they rationalize away their own blame or responsibility. Arguing with a dyslogic student is futile; he will always have the last word.

The most distressing social affect of the dyslogic syndrome is the student's choice of friends or dating partners. Dyslogic young people are especially vulnerable to manipulative and exploitive persons. Because they cannot see consequences in true perspective, dyslogics are open to being used and exploited. I have counseled numerous dyslogic girls who were duped by manipulative men. It is tragic to see pregnancy, venereal disease, young divorce, or heavy financial liability become reality for adolescents who cannot see what is happening in true perspective. Dyslogics usually defend their social partners fiercely, to the point of running away from school or home if forced to choose between traditional standards or those of their nonconformist group. It is a mistake to issue ultimatums to dyslogics. This maneuver usually backfires with the young person taking the opposite side of the issue, even if it means leaving home or school to defend what he believes to be true.

The important point is that the dyslogic syndrome is not dyslexia. Some dyslexics are also dyslogic, but most are not. However, most hyperkinetics are dyslogic. Teachers must be careful not to mistake one syndrome for the other. Unless these children are dealt with early, their adolescent and adult lives hold little hope for traditional success.

Checklist for Hyperkinetic Syndrome

_____Independent Nature

_____Repulsed by cuddling or caressing, beginning in infancy
_____Walked very early
_____Did not go through usual creeping/crawling stages

_____Uncooperative in group situations

_____Self-centered; demands his own way

_____Volatile temper when restricted or denied

_____Oriented toward the present; a "now person;" demands immediate satisfaction

_____Excellent coordination in running, climbing, walking

_____Hyperactivity

_____Incessant handling, exploring, poking into things; usually destructive

_____Instantly reacts to outside stimulus (changes in noise level, temperature, odors, movement, etc.)

_____Extremely restless; compulsive moving about

_____Constantly noisy and disruptive; cannot keep still when demanded

_____Short attention span; poor listening habits; cannot attend more than two or three minutes at a time

_____Antisocial Behavior

_____Unpopular with peers and adults; has reputation of "being a pest"

_____Intimidating, domineering, aggressive; does not respond to lectures on good manners

_____Frequent tantrums; often violent toward whoever denies his wishes

_____Must have own way at any cost; manipulative; bullying in social situations

_____Frequent strong changes of mood; high one day, low the next

_____Easily excitable in group situations; reacts to pressures others hardly perceive

_____High Anxiety Level

_____Constantly in conflict with environment

_____Volatile frustration tendency: set off by the least provocation; younger hyperkinetics cry often; older may sulk and brood; habitually shouts and screams when frustrated

_____Habituated to compulsive mannerisms: nervous tics; hair pulling; knuckle cracking; tongue sucking; massaging of genitals (masturbation); nose picking

_____Sleeps very lightly and fitfully

_____Frequent nightmares, often not remembered next day

_____Cannot stay at table to finish a meal; demands numerous snacks during the day; develops ravenous appetite at odd times

_____Extremely sensitive to criticism; claims "everyone picks on me"

_____Easily excitable in group situations; reacts to pressures others hardly perceive

_____Intelligence Level

_____Above average, often superior mental capacity in childhood; tends to drop in adolescence and adulthood

_____Delinquent Behavior
    _____Tendency toward conflict with civil authority; adolescent behavior often degenerates into misdemeanor or felony charges
    _____Frequently destructive; assaults property or persons when he feels cornered; poor judgment (dyslogic)

_____Scholastic Achievement
    _____Poor academic record; chronic failure pattern; cannot maintain good work output over extended grading periods
    _____Fails to master concepts and skills because of fragmented attention and poor work habits

Distinguishing Dyslexia from Faulty Vision

A rather obvious learning problem has gone unrecognized as such by many classroom teachers and diagnosticians. A substantial number of underachievers who are regarded as perceptually impaired are actually victims of faulty vision. A cluster of problems related to poor eye muscle control, or to erratic functioning of the visual system, frequently is mistaken for dyslexia. Children with these visual defects are sometimes given a clean bill of health by vision specialists who may misinterpret the responses poor readers give to standard tests for vision. Contributing to this diagnostic problem is the fact that disabled learners usually do not volunteer information about how they see. In fact, children with vision deficiencies which contribute to school failure are seldom aware that their vision is abnormal. When such problems as double vision, alternate suppression ("things blink on and off" on the page), or inability to focus properly are detected after years of struggling to read, the student frequently replies, "No one ever asked me about it before." What the child means is that when he has had an eye examination, the examiner did not ask specifically: "Do things blink on and off when you look at a page?" This rather obvious explanation illustrates the need for adults to be thorough and complete in communicating with children who are not doing well in school.

An astonishing pattern has emerged in the evaluation of several hundred students of all ages at our learning center. Sixty-five percent of the underachievers we have diagnosed have required visual correction before effective remediation of learning problems could be attempted.[3] Yet a majority of these students registered 20/20 to 20/30 acuity on

---

[3] Unpublished research findings of the staff of Jordan-Adams Learning Center, 1968-1976.

the Snellen visual standard. These young people had passed vision screening tests at school, and more than half had been evaluated by vision specialists who observed no significant problem. Still, the students could not "see" well enough to succeed in close work.

In studying these puzzling findings carefully, we discovered the key. The general vision of these students was good. They were capable of controlling vision long enough to pass the rather brief tests done by most doctors. The critical factor overlooked by most professionals for many years has been *sustained* visual control. It is relatively unimportant what acuity level a child achieves on a brief Snellen-based examination. The crucial question is how long can he maintain effective control in sustained classwork when seated at his desk.

During the past ten years more and more attention has been turned to the vision of underachievers (see reading list at end of this chapter). Intense controversy exists between two professional groups, optometrists and ophthalmologists. Learning specialists and classroom teachers stand between these conflicting points of view. During the past decade I have found optometry to be increasingly open and attuned to the non-medical daily classroom problems children experience in visual control. Optometrists are rapidly becoming expert in recognizing the non-medical problems we see in poor achievers. Recently educated optometrists have had three to four years of clinical experience with children in school settings learning to identify the visual control problems that frustrate sustained desk work. Optometrists do not deal with medicine, but they are trained to recognize medical problems which they refer to ophthalmologists for treatment. The well-trained optometrist has become a specialist in school vision. He understands the binocular problems and visual difficulties we see in most instances of classroom failure.

To understand the point of view of today's optometrists in relation to school vision, you should read *Vision and Learning Disability*.[4] This anthology discusses in simple terms newly recognized factors which produce stress and failure for so many dyslexic children. A major point of difference between ophthalmology and optometry revolves around the concept of dyslexia. It is absolutely true that visual training and/or glasses cannot "cure" dyslexia, as ophthalmology rightly insists. Classroom teachers must understand this point. Most disabled learners prove to have two problems that interact to disrupt classroom learning. Poor vision is not the same as dyslexia. The two syndromes are probably unrelated, although no one has yet explained why a much higher in-

---

[4] T. N. Greenstein, editor, *Vision and Learning Disability,* American Optometric Association, 7000 Chippewa Street, St. Louis, Missouri, 63119, 1976.

cidence of poor vision is found in learning disabled children when we go beyond the old Snellen standard of 20/20 vision. Correcting a dyslexic child's poor eyesight does not solve his learning disability. However, a child must see well before remediation of his other problems can be accomplished. Optometrists are developing excellent diagnostic techniques to recognize the visual dilemmas of problem learners.

Appendix C presents a simple test for identifying frustrating vision defects in classroom performance. It is not difficult for teachers to recognize symptoms of poor vision and how they differ from other learning problems. The essential factor in identifying these patterns is to keep in mind the work space of the classroom student. It makes virtually no difference how well a child can see across the room (far point). Only a small part of the school day is spent concentrating his vision across the room. Nearsighted (myopic) students come under stress in copying from the chalkboard, but this constitutes only a small part of the school day. The most important factor is how well a child can see when he sits up straight in his chair with both feet on the floor for sustained periods of time. Near point vision is our chief classroom concern, and this area of eyesight has been given almost no attention by most vision specialists.

A student's school day is spent visually between his fingertips and elbow. By extending your writing hand, you can find your own near visual range where most of your desk work is done. With your arm fully extended, your desk top would correspond with the area between your fingertips and elbow. If your arm is tilted up with the elbow resting on the desk near your waist, your reading material would be about where your wristwatch band lies on your arm. Nearsighted students hold their materials closer, while farsighted students hold their books further out. Most of the school day is spent visually within this very limited range. If the student cannot keep print in clear, stable focus between his fingertips and elbow, he cannot cope with the hours of near point concentration expected by his teachers.

The Jordan Vision Screening Test (JVST) is presented in Appendix C. This simplified screening procedure has proved easy and effective in letting classroom teachers screen the visual behaviors of their low achieving students. Certain earmarks of poor classroom vision are quickly identified by following Checklists 1, 2, 3, and 4 on the JVST Scoresheet.

Test 1. Convergence at Near Point.   You can understand the purpose of this simple test by finding your own near point of convergence. Hold a target (pencil or ball-point pen) at arm's length and slowly move it inward toward your nose. Stop the target the moment it begins to blur. On your own outstretched arm note where your blur point is (near your wrist, midway to your elbow, at your elbow, etc.). If you are farsighted, the target will blur quickly, possibly beyond your fingertips. If the target blurs beyond your extended wrist, you are probably wearing bifocals or reading glasses. Without corrective lenses you could not read smaller print. You would hold a book or newspaper at a distance for sustained reading. If you are nearsighted, the target will blur beyond your wrist but will be clear near your nose. For comfortable sustained reading, you should be able to keep the target in clear focus indefinitely at eight inches from your nose.

In doing this convergence test with poor readers, underachievers, and special students, you will be surprised how many cannot achieve or hold near point convergence. If corrective help is not possible for certain students, poor convergence can be by-passed with a large magnifying lens on a handle. Many remedial classes have a supply of magnifiers, either lenses on handles or page-sized plastic sheets that magnify the whole page. These are temporary aids, certainly not intended to correct a student's focus problem, but they will extend his focus time long enough to let him read passages he would otherwise refuse.

Test 2. Target Pursuit at Near Point.   The examiner's guide (see Appendix C) describes how to administer this simple test. Its significance is that students who cannot track (pursue) slowly moving targets usually cannot keep their place in reading. They constantly skip words or parts of words. They often drop whole lines, sometimes two or three lines at a time, as they make the return sweep in sustained reading. They miscall familiar words from one line to the next because their visual field constantly changes. The eye movements you observe in Test 2 correspond closely with the student's saccadic movements during reading (see Glossary).

Primary teachers have always helped beginner pupils learn to track in reading by giving each child a card marker. Marking in beginning reading is essential for immature visual systems that cannot keep the place unaided. Many older students must also use a marker to read successfully. Those who do poorly on Test 2 invariably need to mark in sustained text reading.

Unfortunately, most older students have been shamed by well-meaning adults for using a finger or marker in reading. Teachers traditionally discourage physical marking beyond second grade. Most teachers believe it their duty to press immature pupils to "grow up." Marking becomes a stigma. In many elementary classrooms it is expressly forbidden. There is a high correlation between discipline problems and taking away the markers too soon. If a frustrated child must mark to keep the place but is forbidden to do so, he has no way of coping with the saccadic demands of sustained reading. Taking away the marker too soon creates many more problems than teachers realize.

Not only must you let poor readers mark, you must actually teach certain ones to do so. Older students who cannot track (pursue) the target need to mark. If they are too self-conscious to use a card beneath each line, they usually can learn to follow their index finger, punching or sweeping each word as it is decoded. I have seen many adolescents and young adults self-consciously punch with a pencil eraser, or lay a pocket comb beneath lines of print. Some older students prefer to use the left thumb above the line, punching each word or syllable with the thumb above instead of with a finger beneath. It does not matter how they mark so long as they do so effectively. Many poor readers eventually develop smooth enough binocular control to discontinue marking, except occasionally when they work with difficult material. Some must use a marker all their lives. This should not be a matter of concern. The point is to help students read, not fuss about whether they mark.

We have observed an interesting result of marking on standardized test scores. Students who do poorly on the Jordan Vision Screening Test cannot handle the smaller print of most standardized achievement tests. We have seen significant increases in scores just by having these students use a card marker on the comprehension passages. This provides more stable visual structure than they can achieve on their own with unaided vision. These students do not read faster with a marker, but they identify significant information more efficiently. Weary readers are often rewarded with higher standardized scores with the added structure of marking.

Test 3. Saccadic Control in Oral Reading.　The most direct way to observe eye control for reading is to listen to a student read aloud from a selection at his Instructional Level. As you know, the Instructional Level is from one to two years below the Frustration Level. Any score obtained on a reading test is the student's Frustration Level, his peak performance level. He cannot possibly do sustained class work at this score point. For daily instruction and practice, you must subtract a year or more from his test scores. Oral reading should be done approximately two years below his reading score.

Saccadic control refers to the eye movements we expect to see in efficient reading. This involves binocular vision. The Snellen vision test is based upon monocular vision. One eye is covered (occluded) while the student reads with one eye only, then the other eye is occluded. The Snellen score is computed with the eyes used separately, not together. For many years educators have accepted this visual appraisal without question. But monocular vision has almost no relationship to classroom production. In reading and writing the student must use both eyes simultaneously (binocular vision). The Jordan Vision Screening Test helps you identify the students who cannot do so adequately. Reading proficiency is built upon binocular skill, except for those instances when one eye suppresses (shuts off) altogether. For efficient reading, it is essential that certain eye movement patterns exist.

Saccadic control begins with near point convergence. You have already found your own near point of convergence. Each student is expected to be able to converge, or bring his eyes together upon the same point of focus. The key to efficient reading is being able to hold convergence as the eyes swiftly "hop" from one focus point to the next along the line of print. Saccadic movement is actually a series of very rapid movements. The right eye moves first, quickly leading (finding the new focus point), then stopping. Instantly the left eye moves to that new point of focus and the two images converge into a clear single image, allowing the brain to "take a picture" of the visual field. You will find most of your poor readers unable to achieve or maintain this smooth saccadic rhythm. When binocular control is weak or irregular, as we find it to be in a majority of problem students, it is impossible for efficient saccadic rhythm to be achieved. Frustration rapidly builds toward the exploding point.

Using a marker helps students stabilize poor binocular control up to a point. Most readers with poor saccadic rhythm will always be slow, plodding, jerky readers. They do not respond well to speed reading techniques, as a rule. Many of them must accept this factor as a life-long limitation, but it need not keep them from becoming good readers at a slow pace. This is especially true of dyslexics.

Test 4. Convergence Control in Handwriting.   Classroom teachers have always seen certain students with very awkward pencil grip in writing. Fussing, scolding, lecturing, and shaming have not changed this peculiar pencil grip in these students. Many right-handed students clutch the pencil with the point back under the hand as left-handed students do. This awkward grip is usually related to faulty binocular vision as outlined on the Jordan Vision Screening Test.

When binocular irregularity exists, certain distinguishing earmarks will be seen in the student's writing. Page 151 presents the writing of a girl who scored poorly on the JVST. Her near point of convergence

TEST IX   5.6   + 37
G.E. 5.6

1. tonight
2. street
3. football
4. cool
5. talk
6. stone
7. race
8. spined   spend
9. lunch
10. soap
11. block
12. drive
13. across
14. meet
15. above
16. wait
17. mouth
18. such
19. bought
20. lovely
21. front
22. together
21. farther
22. basket
23. hammer

was twelve inches (between her wrist and elbow); she could not track
the target all the way around the circle, and her oral reading was choppy
with many words skipped. In writing, she alternately leaned very close
to the paper or leaned to one side and peered sideways under her pencil

hand. As you examine her spelling test (see page 149), you will note the ragged, zig-zag left margin. In numbering the lines for the test, her eyes became exhausted before I began pronouncing the words. Number 18 shows the "jump" toward the right which is characteristic of this binocular deficiency. Her visual control was depleted by the time I began the words. As her visual stress mounted, the left margin became increasingly ragged. In examining a variety of student papers, you will often see columns migrate toward the lower right corner of the sheet or zig-zag widely. These are usually symptoms of poor visual control.

Horizontal writing also reveals the binocular problems we find associated with poor saccadic rhythm. The following is an example from a dyslexic child. You will note the uneven horizontal spacing. Some of the symbols are bunched close together; then suddenly wide gaps appear between symbols. This bunch/gap pattern is usually found when students skip words or syllables as they read.

ABCD EfG Hi j Klmnopq
rstu vwxyz

1 2 34 56 78910 111213 141516
17 18 19 20

When these visual patterns exist, teachers encounter behavior problems in the classroom. After all, if a child cannot maintain clear focus, if he constantly loses the place, if his eyes quickly become tired and uncomfortable, and if handwriting produces immediate visual stress, what else is he to do but fidget and become restless and bored? We have identified a behavior syndrome that usually indicates visual stress in students. Of course there are exceptions to this generalization. Not all fidgety students have poor eyesight. Allergies, skin rash, hyperactivity, low blood sugar, or other physical problems might be involved. However, a majority of the students who fit the following pattern manifest significant problems with sustained near vision:

_____Does not like to get busy with reading or writing tasks
_____Appears to "dawdle" during work time; wastes time for no apparent reason
_____Constantly creates distractions for classmates
_____Habitually misplaces pencil, workbook, or work materials
_____"Can't remember" assignments

_____Seldom finishes work during allotted time; must take work home to finish

_____Makes chronic excuses for not doing assignments

_____Becomes fascinated for long periods in nonreading or nonwriting activities

_____Has reputation for being lazy; adults say: "You could do better if you would try"

_____Fidgets and squirms during study time

_____Is constantly out of seat to sharpen pencil or do some irrelevant task

_____Habitually bids for teacher's attention during study time

_____Is always aware of time, constantly hoping bell will ring or study period will be over

_____Frequently complains of "not feeling well" during study time

Making Referrals.   Teachers are often on the spot about making referrals when problems are identified in the classroom. Many school districts have strict policies which limit or forbid classroom teachers from making referrals. Schools with special service departments usually require teachers to follow a chain of command instead of going directly to parents about suspected or observed problems. Often the school nurse must be consulted when poor vision, hearing, or other health factors are suspected. In many districts the nursing staff refers only to medical doctors (ophthalmologists) but not to optometrists. The classroom teacher is often frustrated to have vision referrals come back with the crisp note: "This child has 20/20 vision. There is no problem with his vision." Yet the child continues to manifest the symptoms I have discussed.

Sometimes it is impossible for teachers to see problems solved for certain students. I have taught a number of students for whom help was not available. In such circumstances the teacher must do her best to bypass the problems as much as possible. Using a marker or magnifier for reading usually helps to bypass binocular irregularities or farsightedness. Using the largest print possible will reduce stress to a certain degree. If outside help is not available, the teacher must help the student understand his limitations and teach him whatever bypass techniques she can devise.

In making referrals the first step should be to determine the most reliable sources of help within your community. When vision care is involved, you should feel free to call the receptionists of various optometrists and ophthalmologists and ask specific questions regarding the doctor's diagnosis. You should ask whether he tests specifically for binocular irregularities: Does he spend time checking near point of convergence, amplitude of accommodation, target pursuits, and phoric posture? Does the doctor ask the child to read aloud from a school textbook and do some handwriting in his presence? Does the doctor test for eye/hand coordination or right/left dominance? If the answer is no, or if you receive vague or evasive replies, you should not refer students to that doctor on the basis of the Jordan Vision Screening Test checklists. This pattern calls for a specialist who works with these important aspects of classroom vision. Recently educated optometrists are prepared to correct these visual problems. Some ophthalmologists recognize the problems and refer patients to clinics for orthoptic training. Before sending parents to the eye doctor, you should determine whether your community has the kind of service these students need.

References for Further Reading

1. Anapolle, Louis. "Vision Problems in Developmental Dyslexia." *Journal of Learning Disabilities* 4 (February 1971): 77-83.

2. Apell, Richard J. "Nearpoint Visual Acuity." *Journal of the American Optometric Association* 44 (February 1973): 168-170.

3. Behrmann, Polly. "Is Your Child Ready for School?" *Journal of Learning Disabilities* 5 (May 1972): 291-294.

4. Bing, Lois. "Vision and the 'Right to Read' Effort." *Journal of Learning Disabilities* 5 (December 1972): 626-630.

5. Bishop, Virginia E. *Teaching the Visually Limited Child.* Springfield, Illinois: Charles C. Thomas, 1971.

6. Bizzi, Emilo. "The Coordination of Eye-Head Movements." *Scientific American* 231 (October 1974): 100-106.

7. Breslauer, Ann H., *et al.* "A Visual-Perceptual Training Program." *Academic Therapy Quarterly* 11 (Spring 1976): 321-334.

8. Brod, Nathan, and Hamilton, David. "Binocularity and Reading." *Journal of Learning Disabilities* 6 (November 1973): 574-576.

9. Cantwell, Dennis P., ed. *The Hyperactive Child.* New York: Spectrum Publications, Inc., 1975.

10. Coleman, Howard M. "The West Warwick Visual Perception Study—Part I." *Journal of the American Optometric Association* 43 (April 1972): 452-462.

11. _____. "The West Warwick Visual Perception Study—Part II." *Journal of the American Optometric Association* 43 (May 1972): 532-543.

12. Coleman, Howard M. "Vision Screening of Children in School Health and Medical Programs." *Journal of the American Optometric Association* 45 (May 1974): 575-580.

13. Cook, Virgil L. "Nystagmic Children—Some Case Reports." *Academic Therapy Quarterly* 11 (Summer 1976): 389-392.

14. Cott, Allan. "Megavitamins: The Orthomolecular Approach to Behavioral Disorders and Learning Disabilities." *Academic Therapy Quarterly* 7 (Spring 1972): 245-248.

15. Crook, William G. *Can Your Child Read? Is He Hyperactive?* Jackson, Tennessee: Pedicenter Press, 1975.

16. Evans, J. R., and Efron, Marvin. "Incidence of Lateral Phoria among SLD Children." *Academic Therapy Quarterly* 11 (Summer 1976): 431-433.

17. Faigel, H. C. "The Medical Needs of NH Adolescents." *Helping the Adolescent with the Hidden Handicap.* Los Angeles: California Association for Neurologically Handicapped Children, 1970, pp. 25-28.

18. Fitzpatrick, John P., and Housen, David W. "The Relationship between Classroom Visual Fatigue and Academic Achievement in Elementary School Children." *Journal of the American Optometric Association* 44 (August 1973): 812-823.

19. Flex, Nathan. "The Eye and Learning Disabilities." *Journal of the American Optometric Association* 43 (June 1972): 612-617.

20. Friedman, Nathan. "Is Reading Disability a Fusional Dysfunction?—Part I." *Journal of the American Optometric Association* 45 (May 1974): 619-622.

21. _____. "Specific Visual Fixation Stress and Motor-Learning Difficulty—Part II." *Journal of the American Optometric Association* 43 (February 1972): 166-173.

22. Friedenberg, Harold L. "Visual Skills Testing as a Diagnostic Aid in Learning Disabilities." *Journal of the American Optometric Association* 44 (February 1973): 145-146.

23. Galente, Margaret B. "Cumulative Minor Deficits: A Longitudinal Study of the Relation of Physical Factors to School Achievement." *Journal of Learning Disabilities* 5 (February 1972): 75-80.

24. Giardina, Teresa. "Help for the Hyperactive and Distractible Child." *Academic Therapy Quarterly* 6 (Spring 1971): 313-316.

25. Goldstein, K. M., *et al.* "Family Patterns and the School Performance of Emotionally Disturbed Boys." *Journal of Learning Disabilities* 3 (January 1970): 10-15.

26. Goleman, Daniel. "A New Computer Test of the Brain." *Psychology Today* 9 (May 1976): 44-48.

27. Goodfriend, Ronnie S. *Power in Perception for the Young Child: A Comprehensive Program for the Development of Prereading Visual Perceptual Skills.* New York: Teachers College Press, 1972.

28. Griffin, Donald C. "Saccades as Related to Reading Disorders." *Journal of Learning Disabilities* 7 (May 1974): 310-316.

29. Grinspoon, Lester, and Singer, Susan B. "Amphetamines in the Treatment of Hyperkinetic Children." *Harvard Educational Review* 43 (November 1973): 515-555.

30. Groffman, S. "Experimental Test of Visual Closure." *Journal of the American Optometric Association* 43 (October 1972): 1156-1161.

31. Gunderson, B. V. "Diagnosis of Learning Disabilities: The Team Approach." *Journal of Learning Disabilities* 4 (February 1971): 107-113.

32. Haslam, R.N.A., and Valletutti, P. J. *Medical Problems in the Classroom: the Teacher's Role in Diagnosis and Management.* Baltimore: University Park Press, 1975.

33. Hawley, Clyde, and Buckley, Robert. "Food Dyes and Hyperkinetic Children." *Academic Therapy Quarterly* 10 (Fall 1974): 27-32.

34. Ingram, T.T.S. "The Early Recognition of Handicaps in Childhood." *Journal of Learning Disabilities* 2 (May 1969): 252-255.

35. John, E. Roy. "How the Brain Works—A New Theory." *Psychology Today* 9 (May 1976): 48-52.

36. Kane, Martin. "Perception—the Phenomenon of Figure-Ground." *Journal of the American Optometric Association* 44 (February 1973): 171-178.

37. Kaufman, Lloyd. *Sight and Mind: An Introduction to Visual Perception.* New York: Oxford University Press, 1974.

38. Keith, L. G., *et al.* "Visual Acuity Testing in Young Children." *British Journal of Ophthalmology* 43 (1972): 1191-1202.

39. Kelly, George R. "Group Perceptual Screening at First Grade Level." *Journal of Learning Disabilities* 3 (December 1970): 640-644.

40. Kirk, Samuel A., and Elkins, John. "Identifying Developmental Discrepancies at the Preschool Level." *Journal of Learning Disabilities* 8 (August/September 1975): 417-419.

41. Knights, R. M., and Hinton, G. G. "Minimal Brain Dysfunction: Clinical and Psychological Test Characteristics." *Academic Therapy Quarterly* 4 (Summer 1969): 265-273.

42. Krill, Alex E. "Reading Retardation: Pertinent Information for the Ophthalmologist, Part I." *Ophthalmology Digest* (August 1972): 9-16.

43. Krippner, Stanley. "On Research in Visual Training and Reading Disability." *Journal of Learning Disabilities* 4 (February 1971): 66-76.

44. Magdol, Miriam S. *Perceptual Training in the Kindergarten.* San Rafael, California: Academic Therapy Publications, 1971.

45. McKee, Gordon W. "Vision Screening of Preschool and School Age Children: the Need for Re-evaluation." *Journal of the American Optometric Association* 43 (September 1972): 1062-1073.

46. Millman, H. L. "Minimal Brain Dysfunction in Children: Evaluation and Treatment." *Journal of Learning Disabilities* 3 (February 1970): 89-99.

47. Oppenheimer, Jess. "All about Me." *Journal of Learning Disabilities* 5 (August/September 1972): 408-422.

48. Page, John G., *et al.* "Pemoline (Cylert) in the Treatment of Childhood Hyperkinesis." *Journal of Learning Disabilities* 7 (October 1974): 498-503.

49. Park, G. E. "Ophthalmological Aspects of Learning Disabilities." *Journal of Learning Disabilities* 2 (April 1969): 189-198.

50. Peiser, Irving J. "Vision and Learning Disabilities." *Journal of the American Optometric Association* 43 (February 1972): 152-159.

51. Pierce, John R. "A Clinical Model for Specifying Relationships between Vision Function Problems and Academic Underachievement." *Journal of the American Optometric Association* 44 (February 1973): 152-156.

52. Piggott, Leonard R., *et al.* "Stressful School Work: An Agent of EEG Deterioration." *Journal of Learning Disabilities* 5 (February 1972): 61-67.

53. Powers, Hugh W. S., Jr. "Dietary Measures to Improve Behavior and Achievement." *Academic Therapy Quarterly* 9 (Winter 1973-74): 203-214.

54. Renshaw, Domeena C. *The Hyperactive Child.* Chicago: Nelson-Hall, 1974.

55. Rosenstein, Soloman N. "Dentition—Significant Abnormalities." *Journal of Learning Disabilities* 9 (April 1976): 225-226.

56. Rosner, Jerome, *et al.* "Optometry and Learning Disabilities." *Journal of the American Optometric Association* 45 (May 1974): 561-569.

57. Rosner, Jerome. *Two Developmental Training Devices.* San Rafael, California: Academic Therapy Publications, 1971.

58. ———. "Visual Analysis Training with Preschool Children." *Journal of the American Optometric Association* 45 (May 1974): 584-591.

59. Russell, Elbert W., *et al. Assessment of Brain Damage: A Neuropsychological Key Approach.* New York: Wiley-Interscience, 1970.

60. Schain, Richard J. "Neurological Diagnosis in Children with Learning Disabilities." *Academic Therapy Quarterly* 7 (Winter 1971-72): 139-147.

61. Schnitker, Max. *The Teacher's Guide to the Brain and Learning.* San Rafael, California: Academic Therapy Publications, 1972.

62. Schuell, Hildred. *Aphasia Theory and Therapy.* Baltimore: University Park Press, 1974.

63. Sherman, Arnold. "Relating Vision Disorders to Learning Disability." *Journal of the American Optometric Association* 44 (February 1973): 140-141.

64. Stephenson, Wayland. "Neurological Dysfunctions." *Diagnosis of Learning Difficulties.* Edited by John A.R. Wilson. New York: McGraw-Hill Book Co., 1971, pp. 109-134.

65. Swanson, William L. "Optometric Vision Therapy—How Successful Is It in the Treatment of Learning Disorders?" *Journal of Learning Disabilities* 5 (May 1972): 285-290.

66. Tarnopol, Lester. "Delinquency and Minimal Brain Dysfunction." *Journal of Learning Disabilities* 3 (April 1970): 200-207.

67. Tymchuk, A. J., *et al.* "The Behavioral Significance of Differing EEG Abnormalities in Children with Learning and/or Behavior Problems." *Journal of Learning Disabilities* 3 (November 1970): 547-551.

68. Van Donge, N. W. "Visual Problems in the Classroom." *Diagnosis of Learning Difficulties.* Edited by John A.R. Wilson. New York: McGraw-Hill Book Co., 1971, pp. 37-60.

69. von Hilshimer, George. *Allergy, Toxins and the Learning Disabled Child.* San Rafael, California: Academic Therapy Publications, 1974.

70. _____. *How to Live with Your Special Child: A Handbook for Behavior Change.* Washington, D.C.: Acropolis Books, 1970.

71. Weintraub, Samuel. *Vision-Visual Discrimination.* International Reading Association and ERIC/CRIER, 1973.

72. Wilson, W. Keith, and Wold, Robert M. "A Report on Vision Screening in the Schools." *Academic Therapy Quarterly* 8 (Winter 1972-73): 155-166.

73. Woodruff, M. E. "The Visually 'At Risk' Child." *Journal of the American Optometric Association* 44 (February 1973): 130-134.

74. Wunderlich, Ray C. *Allergy, Brains, and Children Coping.* St. Petersburg, Florida: Johnny Reads, Inc., 1973.

75. _____. "Biosocial Factors in the Child with School Problems." *Academic Therapy Quarterly* 10 (Summer 1975): 389-399.

76. _____. "Hyperkinetic Disease." *Academic Therapy Quarterly* 5 (Winter 1969-70): 99-108.

JOST—Jordan Oral Screening Test

Administering the JOST

The examiner should give the student a separate score sheet. The student's errors should never be marked on the same copy from which he is reading. As the student reads aloud, the examiner makes quick notations of mispronunciations, substitutions, reversals, failure to perceive minimal cues, or other types of reading errors. This is best done by writing down exactly what the student says, as nearly as the error can be duplicated by the examiner. It is important that these notes be made so an accurate analysis for dyslexic factors can be done at a later time. It is often helpful to record the number of correct responses at each level. The examiner can quickly jot down the number of correct responses on the blank space before each numeral 10, the last word in each column.

Do not expect a struggling reader to say "Skip" when he comes to a word he cannot decode. The examiner can usually tell from the reader's manner whether his vision has skipped (failed to see) a word, or whether he has given up and gone on to another item. It is intensely frustrating to dyslexics to have examiners nag about giving stereotyped responses, such as remembering to say "Skip." Be prepared to interpret the reader's effort rather than depending upon him to give cues whenever he leaves out difficult items.

The examiner should look for patterns of errors. For example, the student may not know the sound of *si* and *ci* in such words *delicious* (Level Five), *graciously* (Level Six), *commercially* and *impressionable* (Level Eight). This would be a teaching cue, indicating a specific phonetic generalization the student has never mastered. The words *legion* and *nation* indicate the student's knowledge of the sound of vowels in open syllables. A careful study of the reading mistakes (item analysis) does not take long, and it will give the teacher several specific prescriptions for class assignments to help the student improve his word analysis skills.

The JOST is *not* a timed test in any way. One of the worst possible situations for a dyslexic child is to be under timed pressure while reading or writing. The examiner should make brief notes on the score sheet about unusual slowness or speed. Most students who score below Reading Level 6.0 will be slow readers. The lower the JOST Reading Level score, the slower the decoding process, as a rule.

The JOST is not a standardized instrument. The scores of hundreds of students ranging from Grade Two through Adult have been compared with achievement test scores these students made under timed limitations. The JOST Reading Level score usually predicts the student's comprehension level within a range of six months. For example, if a student scores Reading Level 4.0, his standardized achievement test score in reading comprehension will probably be between 3.7 and 4.3.

The examiner must keep in mind that any test score is the Frustration Level, not the Instruction Level. A rule of thumb is that one to two full years should be subtracted to estimate the student's comfortable Instruction Level where he can read for sustained periods of time with minimum frustration. While this makes remediation seem slow, following this rule allows dyslexic students to gain a sense of confidence. Teachers who plunge poor readers into material that causes frustration lose far more than is gained.

Score Sheet—JOST—Jordan Oral Screening Test

Name_____ Date_____

year   month   day

Grade in School_____ Birth Date_____

year   month   day

Reading Level_____ Age_____

years   months

DIRECTIONS: Read the words aloud. If you come to a word you do not know, say "Skip."

Level One	*Level Two*	*Level Three*	*Level Four*
1. and	1. we	1. same	1. can't
2. up	2. can	2. gave	2. circus
3. but	3. jump	3. suddenly	3. herself
4. so	4. foot	4. rope	4. smart
5. it	5. help	5. heaven	5. platform
6. he	6. baby	6. happened	6. exclaim
7. something	7. mother	7. start	7. understand
8. run	8. play	8. farmer	8. wouldn't
9. me	9. come	9. along	9. street
10. see	10. bark	10. around	10. learn
___	___	___	___

Level Five	*Level Six*	*Level Seven*	*Level Eight*
1. answers	1. examples	1. radiation	1. redundancy
2. silver	2. criticize	2. medicine	2. forfeit
3. careless	3. graciously	3. customarily	3. commercially
4. grave	4. snuggle	4. yearling	4. standardized
5. speaking	5. natural	5. future	5. impressionable
6. already	6. punishment	6. knowledge	6. extraordinary
7. delicious	7. exercise	7. stallion	7. physiology
8. dumpling	8. obey	8. abundance	8. zephyr
9. legion	9. musical	9. accidental	9. environmental
10. nation	10. religion	10. preoccupy	10. intoxicating
___	___	___	___

Note: A perfect score on this page yields Reading Level 8.0, the lower limit of functional literacy.

Level Nine
1. destitution
2. burlesque
3. projectile
4. brogue
5. humiliation
6. supplemental
7. irrelevance
8. ingeniously
9. depreciation
10. intangibly

Level Ten
1. felonious
2. disproportionate
3. antigravity
4. irrepressible
5. instantaneously
6. fiance
7. naive
8. requisition
9. noninflammable
10. countermanded

Level Eleven
1. reprehensibly
2. excruciating
3. xerography
4. ionospheric
5. coalition
6. idiosyncrasy
7. eccentricity
8. envisage
9. affability
10. irrationality

Level Twelve
1. vermifuge
2. avuncular
3. auspiciously
4. antisecessionism
5. verisimilitude
6. disassociation
7. extracurricular
8. iconoclasticism
9. prestidigitation
10. psychosomatic

Level Thirteen
1. unameliorative
2. omnipotence
3. hyperkinesis
4. pseudosophisticate
5. lasciviously
6. hypothyroidism
7. automatism
8. interlocutor
9. irrefragable
10. semiconsciousness

1. Record the number correct at each reading level.
2. Add to find **TOTAL CORRECT.**
3. Insert decimal in ten's place in **TOTAL CORRECT.**
4. This is the JOST Reading Level score.

Example: Reading Level 8.3 would mean eighth year, third month, grade equivalent

Level One_____
Level Two_____
Level Three_____
Level Four_____
Level Five_____
Level Six_____
Level Seven_____
Level Eight_____
Level Nine_____
Level Ten_____
Level Eleven_____
Level Twelve_____
Level Thirteen_____
TOTAL CORRECT_____
Reading Level_____

NOTE: The JOST Reading Level score is the student's peak performance level, the best he can do. This is called the *frustration level.* The *instructional level* begins at least two years below this point. *Leisure reading* will be three or more years below this score.

appendix b

JWST—Jordan Written Screening Test for Specific Reading Disability

Administering the JWST

The Jordan Written Screening Test is intended for use with English-speaking persons having conversational fluency with American English speech. The examiner must be careful to distinguish between total illiteracy and dyslexia. Many persons simply have never learned the alphabet or the fundamentals of reading.

The JWST is designed for right-handedness because a majority of persons are right-handed. Left-handed (sinistral) writers, however, are not penalized by this screening test. The examiner should take into account the usual problems in writing that are experienced by left-handed students in a right-handed culture. The comments about backward hand motions do not apply to left-handed writers, as a rule. The sole criterion for the left-handed student should be legibility when there is no evidence of faulty muscle control.

The JWST is not intended to yield a concrete scale or sequence of scores. The test is designed to show tendencies toward symbol confusion and disorientation. When the testing is finished, the examiner should fill in the Dyslexia Profile on the student's book while the child's behavior is still freshly in mind. If only a few dyslexic characteristics are indicated by the overall performance, then the student would not be termed dyslexic. If a definite cluster of symptoms is clearly revealed by the test responses, and the student clearly confuses letters, words, numerals, and sequence, then he can safely be designated as dyslexic.

Mental ability and educational background are important factors in determining dyslexia. An actual IQ score is not essential, but a general estimate of low, average, or high intelligence needs to be indicated. Low mental ability often produces reading errors similar to dyslexia. Persons with actual mental ability below an IQ of 80 usually display slowness, as well as symbol confusion, difficulty with spelling, and problems in following sequence.

It is essential that the source of any intelligence scores be known; otherwise they should be disregarded. Group IQ tests which require reading ability cannot yield valid mental ability estimates for poor readers. Such tests are first of all reading tests. Persons reading below grade level cannot comprehend group IQ test items well enough to make valid responses to the test items. If the JOST Reading Level score is more than one full year below the student's grade placement, then any IQ score obtained from a timed group test should be disregarded.

Group Test Items (1–14)

Tests 1 through 14 may be administered to small groups of five or six students, depending upon the facilities available for testing. Students should not be crowded together. The test monitor or examiner must be able to watch the hand movements of each student during the writing activities. If the JWST is administered to small groups, care must be taken that no student picks up cues from another's paper. If dyslexia is to be determined, the examiner must be sure that a valid individual response is being recorded.

Test 1—Write the Alphabet

If the student does not know how to write the alphabet, he may say it while the examiner writes down his oral response. It does not matter if the student prints or writes cursive style. The examiner should make no comment unless the student asks how he should write. "Whatever way is most comfortable for you" is all the structure the examiner should give. The point is for the student to make a natural response.

If the student cannot remember which letter comes next, the examiner may say the name of the letter, or write it for the student to see. A note should be made when any kind of assistance is given.

The examiner should be alert for tendencies to write letters backwards or upside down. It is important to observe any backward motions in writing (clockwise strokes on circles; marking from bottom to top).

Test 2—Write your Birthday (month, day, year)

The examiner should write down oral responses of illiterate students. The purpose of this test is to determine how well the student handles sequence, which is an important factor in determining dyslexia. Any tendency to make numerals backward or to mark from the bottom upward should be noted.

Test 3—Write the Days of the Week

Again the examiner should write for an illiterate student. Notes should be made of any kind of memory device used by the student (mumbling a rhyme, humming a song, counting on fingers, tapping the table, going back to the first day each time a new one is named or written).

The purpose of this test is to gather further evidence of difficulty with sequence and chronological order, as well as tendencies to reverse or rotate letters, or to use backward motions in writing.

Auditory dyslexia is indicated by poor spelling of these words, which have been a common element in the student's life. Phonetic spellings are especially significant (Munday, Toosday, Winsday).

Test 4—Write the Months of the Year

It is often necessary to suggest that the student start with January and name the rest of the months. A note should be made if this anchor point is needed to start the student naming the months.

Dyslexics often add spring, winter, fall, summer, Christmas, or other seasonal designations when naming months. The examiner should note any other unusual aspects of the student's response. He should be allowed to use abbreviations or first letters only if he is unable to try to spell out the full names. *This is not a spelling test.* This activity is an estimate of ability to handle sequence and chronological order of common cultural factors.

Test 5—Copy the Story Like It Is on the Chart

This test estimates the student's ability to copy from far point without scrambling the order of letters and words. The test provides a quick estimate of perception of minimal cues, such as paragraph indention, spacing, punctuation marks, and similar words and letters. Dyslexic tendencies to reverse (was for saw), rotate (d for b), perseverate (add extra syllables or letters), or telescope (leave out letters or syllables) will quickly become apparent.

The following story should be printed (cursive style is acceptable for students above Grade Three) on a wall chart or on the chalkboard. The student should sit not closer than ten feet from the chart or board.

Bob and Dan

Bob and Dan saw Sam Watts on
the dock. The three men stopped.
"See the big ship?" asked Sam.
"Sure did," Dan and Bob said.
"Must be a mile long."
Bob and Dan saw Sam was in a
hurry. "Got to run," Sam said.
"See you."
"Sure," said Bob and Dan. "See
you, Sam."

Test 6—Write the Words I Say for You

It is essential that the examiner pronounce these words clearly. Certain American dialects do not pronounce the /r/ sounds, whereas other dialects leave off final sounds. This test may not be valid if given by an examiner who speaks a dialect that is noticeably different from that of his students. If the examiner blurs phonic components of the words the students may not be able to make valid responses in writing.

Most dyslexics are disturbed if the examiner continues talking while the students are trying to write. The examiner must make sure that the students know what each word means, but the examiner should not follow the usual format of spelling tests. It is best if the examiner *does not* say the word, use it in a sentence, and then say the word again while the students are trying to write. When the students know the word, the examiner should then remain silent unless asked to repeat or clarify a meaning.

The test words are arranged so the examiner can quickly scan for dyslexic tendencies. The words are grouped in sets of frequently made errors, which will allow quick evaluation of the written responses.

1. dig	14. pig	27. big
2. ate	15. rode	28. goes
3. play	16. please	29. toes
4. duck	17. buck	30. track
5. party	18. pretty	31. try
6. brown	19. born	32. for
7. barn	20. brand	33. from
8. girl	21. bird	34. stop
9. saw	22. was	35. post
10. kind	23. king	36. slat
11. city	24. cent	37. salt
12. this	25. think	38. how
13. on	26. no	39. who

Test 7—Copy Each Drawing Three Times

This test indicates dysgraphia, which is the inability to control hand movements for legible writing. The examiner should watch for distorted shapes in the student's work. Particularly significant are corners that are not closed, as well as oblong or misshaped circles. Many dysgraphics make "ears" on corners because they cannot control the fine motor movements for correct line production.

Test 8—Write Down Exactly What You Hear Me Say

The purpose of this dictation test is to estimate the student's auditory perception, as well as his skill in associating sounds with symbols. Dyslexic confusion with sounds, as well as tendencies to reverse, rotate, or write in mirror image, will be indicated by the written responses. The examiner should pronounce each item slowly and steadily with approximately one second time lapse between each item. The student is not to begin writing until the examiner has finished pronouncing each set. If necessary, the student's book may need to be turned over while he listens.

As in all dictated tests, it is essential that the examiner's own speech be clear. If the pronunciation is mushy or garbled, the student is at a great disadvantage, being forced to guess at what is said.

     1. b–e–g
     2. m–f–p–l
     3. t–z–c–b

4. one–twenty-one
5. f–t–j–i–h
6. eighteen–forty-five
7. b–v–d–p
8. three–nine–eight–twelve
9. fifty-seven–ninety-six–twenty-one
10. put the tub on top

Note: When using these tests with young children (below Grade Three) the examiner may choose to give fewer items in the longer series. For example, if the pupil is obviously unable to cope with more than three factors in a series, then the longer items may be abbreviated to only three dictation factors.

Test 9—Write the First Letter You Hear in Each Word

This is a test of sound-symbol relationships, as well as of identifying the initial position of these discrete sound elements. Auditory dyslexics have difficulty identifying individual phonic sounds accurately. The examiner should look for a pattern of mistakes which shows that the student does not perceive similar sounds accurately.

1. touch	(t)	6. zephyr	(z)
2. dike	(d)	7. seldom	(s)
3. mark	(m)	8. built	(b)
4. pat	(p)	9. fawn	(f)
5. welt	(w)	10. vixen	(v)

Test 10—Write the Last Letter You Hear in Each Word

1. pelt	(t)	6. hiss	(s) or (ss)
2. hod	(d)	7. fuzz	(z) or (zz)
3. stub	(b)	8. listen	(n) or (cn)
4. riff	(f) or (ff)	9. thrum	(m)
5. rave	(v) or (ve)	10. stir	(r) or (ir)

Test 11—Write the First Two Letters You Hear in Each Word

This is a test of the student's perception of consonant clusters, also called digraphs and blends. Auditory dyslexics have great difficulty identifying the separate parts of consonant clusters.

1. brat	(br)	6. fluke	(fl)
2. slake	(sl)	7. choke	(ch)
3. twine	(tw)	8. shim	(sh)
4. grit	(gr)	9. tripe	(tr)
5. platten	(pl)	10. drouth	(dr)

Test 12—Write the Last Two Letters You Hear in Each Word

1. lurch	(ch)	6. gong	(ng)
2. mush	(sh)	7. booth	(th)
3. smack	(ck)	8. smooth	(th)
4. lisp	(sp)	9. wrist	(st)
5. bard	(rd)	10. slurp	(rp)

Note: The examiner should make a difference in enunciating the hard *th* in "booth" and the soft *th* in "smooth."

Test 13—Mark the Word That Is Like the Word You See on the Card

This test will indicate tendencies to read words backwards, or to perceive letters backwards, upside down, or in transposed positions inside words.

Ten flash cards should be made of uniform size with these words printed in large manuscript letters: barn   tops   silver   trap   must   reverse   sheep   boob   trash   wash

The cards should be shown for a few seconds, usually until the examiner detects a cue that the student feels he knows the word or at least comprehends the letter sequence. If the examiner thinks the student is not concentrating on the task, a simple reminder would be useful: "Be sure you study it carefully." Then the student finds the matching word on his work page. It is not important whether the student can pronounce the words on the cards. The examiner is free to say the words if it is obvious the student cannot read them. The student may see the card several times as he tries to match the form on the page. If this is necessary, a note should be made for future reference. The purpose of this test is to see whether the student can match sequence and position of letters without visual cues.

1.	bran	pran	puar	bnar	narb	uarp	*barn*
2.	spot	tops	*tops*	stop	stob	sbot	tods
3.	sliver	*silver*	vilser	revils	revlis	selvir	verlis
4.	trad	brat	rapt	part	prat	bart	*trap*
5.	tums	tsum	smut	swnt	tsuw	*must*	wnst
6.	severe	esrever	*reverse*	eversen	servere	neverse	nervese
7.	sheeb	speeh	sheed	skeey	*sheep*	speey	peehs
8.	poop	dood	boop	poob	*boob*	doob	doop
9.	tarsh	shraf	farsh	shart	*trash*	frash	shart
10.	mash	sham	*wash*	shaw	whas	hsaw	sahw

Test 14—Mark the Word That Is Like the One You Hear Me Say

It is essential that the examiner pronounce these words clearly. The word "which" must *not* be pronounced "witch" if the student is to hear the /h/ value and mark the correct choice.

1. "which"	1. wish	*which*	witch	with
2. "every"	2. *every*	ever	very	even
3. "shine"	3. chime	shin	*shine*	chin
4. "prior"	4. *prior*	prayer	pry	priory
5. "riot"	5. write	right	rite	*riot*
6. "quit"	6. *quit*	quiet	quite	quid
7. "scorch"	7. scratch	scarce	*scorch*	source
8. "valve"	8. vowel	val	*valve*	value
9. "madge"	9. mash	*madge*	match	mad
10. "singer"	10. sinker	*singer*	sinner	seen

Individual Test Items (15–18)

The following test items must be administered on a one-to-one basis. If other students are to take these tests later, they must not overhear this activity.

Test 15—Repeat Exactly What You Hear Me Say

This test is an estimate of auditory dyslexic tendency to hear and reproduce syllables in the wrong sequence within words (echolalia). These tongue twisters will reveal dyslexic tendencies quickly. The examiner should write down exactly what the student says if a mispronunciation is given. It is usually best to say the phrase again, giving a second or third chance for the student to repeat it correctly. If a correct response is made, the examiner may make a check mark to save time.

It is essential that the examiner be practiced enough to say these phrases without stumbling. This test will be of little value if the examiner does not provide an accurate, clear speech model for the student.

1. olives in vinegar
2. aluminum animal
3. suddenly suspicious
4. curiosity seekers
5. announced candidacy
6. conscientious maneuver

Test 16—Repeat These Sentences Word for Word after I Say Them

The purpose of this test is to estimate the student's ability to recall sequence and order. Auditory dyslexia is also indicated if the student has difficulty pronouncing certain words. The examiner should speak rather slowly in a steady rhythm, making sure the thought units are phrased vocally.

1. Three men — raced down the hill — to the boat — in the river.

2. After dark one night — he gave the money — to his best friend.

Test 17—Repeat These Numbers after You Hear Me Say Them

This test indicates the student's ability to handle several items in a series without visual cues. The examiner should write down what the student says in order to have a record of any scrambled pattern which emerges.

1. 6 – 5 – 4 – 3 – 2 – 7
2. 8 – 9 – 2 – 7 – 5

Test 18—Give a Word That Rhymes with Each Word I Say

The examiner should write down exactly what the student says. Differences in dialect should be allowed, the purpose being to see whether the individual recognizes words that sound very much alike. It is important to remember that this is an oral rhyming test, not a spelling test.

For example, many family groups pronounce *sure* as "shore." If the student gives a rhyming word like "pore" or "yore," this should be accepted as a correct rhyming response to *sure*.

Nonsense responses should not be counted as correct. Many auditory dyslexics can mimic similar words, but do not actually hear rhyming elements. For example, a dyslexic might say "mowd" to rhyme with *crowd*. This is an example of mimicry, not of understanding the function of rhymes. Such a response should not be counted as correct.

1.	take	(make, bake)
2.	hot	(lot, not)
3.	said	(red, head)
4.	seat	(heat, beat)
5.	crowd	(loud, cowed)
6.	station	(nation, isolation)
7.	brother	(mother, other)
8.	preacher	(teacher, creature)
9.	sure	(cure, your)
10.	whistle	(missle, bristle)

JWST—Jordan Written Screening Test

Name_____   Date_____

JOST Reading Level Score_____   Birthdate_____
year   month   day

Highest Grade Completed_____   Age_____
years   months

Estimated Intelligence__ __ __
low average high

Handedness__ __
right left

Dyslexia Profile

	none	moderate	pronounced	severe
Visual Dyslexia	_____	_____	_____	_____
	none	moderate	pronounced	severe
Auditory Dyslexia	_____	_____	_____	_____
	none	moderate	pronounced	severe
Dysgraphia	_____	_____	_____	_____

Visual Dyslexia	*Auditory Dyslexia*	*Dysgraphia*
__ Perceives symbols backward, upside down, in scrambled sequence	__ Does not distinguish separate phonic elements in words	__ Writes letters, words, numerals backward (mirror image)
__ Reverses words, syllables, number units	__ Cannot detect syllables	__ Cannot recall how to write certain symbols
__ Leaves off endings	__ Cannot determine accent	__ Distorts letters or numerals
__ Misreads similar words, letters, numerals	__ Cannot blend word parts into whole word units	__ Has difficulty writing legibly
__ Telescopes in reading	__ Cannot apply simple phonic rules to reading or spelling	__ Uses backward motions in writing certain symbols
__ Perseverates in reading	__ Gives garbled pronunciation to common words (echolalia)	__ Has difficulty copying accurately
__ Cannot recall correct sequence of letters, words, numerals	__ Writes words phonetically	__ Has difficulty copying or tracing simple shapes
__ Has difficulty recalling information in sequence (alphabet, days of week, months of year, sentences, number groups, etc.)	__ Asks speaker to repeat	__ Telescopes in writing
	__ Subvocalizes while reading or writing	__ Perseverates in writing
	__ Erases, marks over habitually while writing	

1. Write the Alphabet

_____

_____

_____

2. Write Your Birthday (month, day, year)

_____

3. Write the Days of the Week

_____

_____

_____

4. Write the Months of the Year

_____

_____

_____

_____

_____

_____

5. Copy the Story Like It Is on the Chart

_____

_____

_____

_____

_____

_____

_____

_____

_____

_____

_____

6. Write the Words I Say for You

1. _____	14. _____	27. _____
2. _____	15. _____	28. _____
3. _____	16. _____	29. _____
4. _____	17. _____	30. _____
5. _____	18. _____	31. _____
6. _____	19. _____	32. _____
7. _____	20. _____	33. _____
8. _____	21. _____	34. _____
9. _____	22. _____	35. _____
10. _____	23. _____	36. _____
11. _____	24. _____	37. _____
12. _____	25. _____	38. _____
13. _____	26. _____	39. _____

7. Copy Each Drawing Three Times

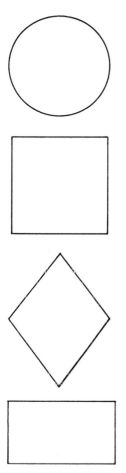

8. Write Down Exactly What You Hear Me Say

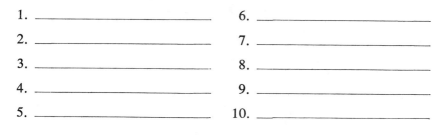

1. _____   6. _____

2. _____   7. _____

3. _____   8. _____

4. _____   9. _____

5. _____   10. _____

_____

9. Write the First Letter You Hear in Each Word

1. _____   6. _____
2. _____   7. _____
3. _____   8. _____
4. _____   9. _____
5. _____   10. _____

10. Write the Last Letter You Hear in Each Word

1. _____   6. _____
2. _____   7. _____
3. _____   8. _____
4. _____   9. _____
5. _____   10. _____

11. Write the First Two Letters You Hear in Each Word

1. _____   6. _____
2. _____   7. _____
3. _____   8. _____
4. _____   9. _____
5. _____   10. _____

12. Write the Last Two Letters You Hear in Each Word

1. _____   6. _____
2. _____   7. _____
3. _____   8. _____
4. _____   9. _____
5. _____   10. _____

13. Mark the Word That Is Like the Word You See on the Card

1.	bran	pran	puar	bnar	narb	uarp	barn
2.	spot	tobs	tops	stop	stob	sbot	tods
3.	sliver	silver	vilser	revils	revlis	selvir	verlis
4.	trad	brat	rapt	part	prat	bart	trap
5.	tums	tsum	smut	swnt	tsuw	must	wnst.
6.	severe	esrever	reverse	eversen	servere	neverse	nervese
7.	sheeb	speeh	sheed	sdeey	sheep	speey	peehs
8.	poop	dood	boop	poob	boob	doob	doop
9.	tarsh	shraf	farsh	shart	trash	frash	sharf
10.	mash	sham	wash	shaw	whas	hsaw	sahw

14. Mark the Word That Is Like The One You Hear Me Say

1.	wish	which	witch	with
2.	every	ever	very	even
3.	chime	shin	shine	chin
4.	prior	prayer	pry	priory
5.	write	right	rite	riot
6.	quit	quiet	quite	quid
7.	scratch	scarce	scorch	source
8.	vowel	val	valve	value
9.	mash	madge	match	mad
10.	sinker	singer	sinner	seen

15. Repeat Exactly What You Hear Me Say

1. _____   _____
2. _____   _____
3. _____   _____
4. _____   _____
5. _____   _____
6. _____   _____

16. Repeat These Sentences Word for Word after I Say Them

1. _____

2. _____

17. Repeat These Numbers after You Hear Me Say Them

    1. _____

    2. _____

18. Give a Word That Rhymes with Each Word I Say

    1. _____   6. _____

    2. _____   7. _____

    3. _____   8. _____

    4. _____   9. _____

    5. _____   10. _____

appendix c

JVST—Jordan Vision Screening Test for Binocular Control for Sustained Reading and Handwriting

Administering the JVST

Test 1—Convergence at Near Point

The examiner sits directly in front of the student, making sure he is on eye level with the student and near enough so their knees almost touch. The student holds out his writing hand with palm turned up and fingers straight. If the student is not too self-conscious, he should lay his arm on top of the examiner's outstretched arm. Starting at the student's fingertips the examiner slowly moves the target (a pencil or ball-point pen) toward the student's nose.

The student is to tell whenever the target goes out of focus, doubles, disappears, or otherwise becomes distorted. The examiner must phrase his questions to fit the language maturity of the student. A young child might say, "It goes all fuzzy," while an older person might say, "It goes out of focus." The wording does not matter so long as the point of the activity is clear.

In this test, the critical distance lies between the student's wrist and elbow. This is why he extends his arm. The examiner's task is to determine whether visual distortion occurs within this area while the student concentrates his vision upon the target. The target can be a pencil, a writing pen, a small flashlight, or any object that presents a contrasting focal spot.

The examiner watches the student's eyes by sighting past the moving target. Major (gross) eye movement tendencies will be obvious. The purpose of this test is to observe more subtle manifestations of faulty binocularity. The examiner must be alert for one eye shifting away from the other, widening of the eyes as the target moves closer, leaning back or to one side, squinting, watering of the eyes, or any look of puzzlement or surprise on the student's face. Often a student will indicate changes in visual clarity by exclaiming, "Wow!" or "Golly!" If this occurs, the examiner should ask the student to explain what happened.

Note: This convergence test *must not* be hurried. Most problems in maintaining convergence do not show up until the eyes have been focused for half a minute or more. A quick test administration usually does not produce the muscle imbalance tendencies which cause visual fatigue during sustained reading and writing in the classroom.

Test 2—Target Pursuit at Near Point

The examiner holds the target at arm's length from the student's face as the student sits back in his chair. The student is instructed to hold his head still and to move only his eyes. If he cannot keep from turning his head to follow the target, he may cup his chin in his hands to hold his head still. The examiner should make a note of this need for help in keeping the head from turning.

As he slowly moves the target in an arc, the examiner closely watches the student's eyes. Faulty eye control causes either or both of the eyes to jump away from the target. The examiner is alert for jerky eye movements, watering of the eyes, squinting, widening of the eyes, or other problems keeping the eyes focused on the slowly moving target. Where faulty convergence is pronounced, the student's eyes will "quiver" or "dance" as the target moves through the arc.

The examiner is alert for such visual problems as blurring, doubling, or disappearing of the target at certain spots throughout the arc. The target should be moved left-to-right through a complete circle, then right-to-left through a circle, then up-and-down, then side-to-side. This routine should continue for half a minute or more to determine how long the student can track the target and keep it in focus.

Students often indicate visual frustration by exclaiming "Hmmmm!" "Wow!" "Man!" or "Golly!" The examiner should ask for an explanation of what is happening when this reaction occurs. Poor muscle balance will cause a student to lean back, forward, or sideways as he tracks the target. He may turn his head instead of his eyes, or he may look at an angle toward the target.

Note: This test *must not* be hurried or rushed. The point is to observe the student's visual control during sustained tracking. This closely resembles the student's eye movements in keeping his place on the line while reading.

Test 3—Saccadic Control in Oral Reading

The examiner follows one copy of text while the student reads aloud from another copy. Children in Grades 1-3 should read from primary material in which the print is large and there is ample white space. Older students should read from smaller print that corresponds to the type size used in their classroom texts, library materials, or remedial reading books.

As the student reads aloud, the examiner is alert for skipping of syllables, word endings, whole words, or even whole sentences. When the student has poor saccadic control, he begins to skip word elements almost immediately because his eyes do not maintain consistent focus along the line. Problems in maintaining saccadics may not become noticeable until the student has read two or more pages. Skipping will cause the student to pause frequently, stop suddenly within words, or back up and re-read words or phrases in order to pick up the lost continuity. As eye muscles become more poorly coordinated, skipping becomes more pronounced. The student begins to mispronounce familiar words. He may correctly say a word on one line, but a few lines later fail to pronounce the same word because its configuration has changed as his eyes skip. Eventually his reading becomes so faulty that he wants to terminate the activity.

The examiner watches for a tendency to mark the place with a finger, thumb, pencil, or some other kind of marker. Some students have developed habits of marking to hold the place, while others have not learned to do so. The examiner makes a note of any aids the student uses to keep his place on the line. It is also important to learn whether the student's teachers permit marking at school. If teachers forbid marking, students with faulty saccadics are at a serious disadvantage.

During oral reading, the examiner looks for other problems in maintaining focus. More serious vision problems cause the student to hold the book to one side, peering sideways instead of straight ahead. The student may say, "My nose gets in the way, so I have to turn my head." Some students hold the book down and look upward to read, as if peering over a pair of glasses. The examiner watches for such habits as holding the book very close, leaning close to the book on the desk, constantly shifting position during reading, or trying to terminate the reading activity. Poor saccadic control produces watering, squinting, or widening of the eyes as the student reads. Many students rub or brush at their eyes while reading.

Sometimes faulty muscle balance causes the eyes to dart constantly about the page. When the student comes to an unknown word, his tendency may be to glance all around the page for clues. In the middle of a word his eyes may jump to a spot several inches from the focal point. This "dance" is characteristic of a frustrating form of muscle imbalance that usually does not show up on standard visual examinations.

The purpose of this oral reading test is to inform the teacher of how long the student can stay with sustained reading in the classroom. If the student does poorly on this test, he cannot do study assignments that require him to concentrate his vision between wrist and elbow for more than five minutes at one sitting. Therefore a twenty- or thirty-minute study task is out of the question without triggering discipline problems.

Test 4—Convergence Control in Handwriting

The examiner gives the student a pencil and a sheet of lined paper. Primary pupils (Grades 1-3) should use wide-line tablet paper. Older students (Grade 4 and above) should write on regular notebook or tablet paper.

The examiner observes how the student grips his pencil for writing. The "normal" writing grip for right-handed students is for the pencil point to protrude between index and middle fingers while the thumb holds the pencil firmly against the index finger. Left-handed writers usually hold the pencil in a similar way, although their grip is turned inward. The examiner must not confuse left-handedness with abnormal grip.

When faulty eye muscle balance exists, or the eyes do not stay aligned properly during sustained near-point vision, one eye or the other will turn away from the focal point. In handwriting, both eyes should be focused upon the pencil point as it moves along the line. As one eye or the other moves away, the student no longer sees the pencil point clearly. In order to keep it in clear focus, he turns the pencil point straight downward, or pulls it back toward his body. Often the hand is made into a fist with the pencil protruding downward under the knuckles. At the same time he may roll his head to one side, or turn the paper at a sharp angle. This combination of abnormal grip, head turning, and/ or paper turning indicates faulty vision.

By taking ample time and talking about what the student sees as he writes, the examiner and student can plot the eye movements along a line of writing. Most students have never before realized that one eye may not track with the other. It often comes as a surprise for them to realize that one eye sees one point on the page while the other eye concentrates on another spot. The examiner must be sure not to worry the student about such eye behavior. If the student expresses anxiety, the examiner must assure him that this is very common. Many people find their eyes doing this sort of thing from time to time. The point is to help the student understand that this is why he has had problems doing certain kinds of school work. Self-understanding usually relieves anxiety.

The examiner also examines the writing for uneven spacing between letters and words. As the eyes jump to new focal points along the line, irregular spacing occurs. The student is so intent upon keeping the pencil point in focus that he fails to control letter and word spacing. Even though the pencil grip may be normal and there may not be any obvious shifting of the eyes, irregular spacing usually indicates deficiencies in maintaining near vision. Faulty binocular control also causes the student to write large letters and numerals. Unusually large, irregularly spaced symbols often signify faulty eye control for handwriting.

Faulty binocular control produces a zig-zag, wobbly left margin as the student makes numeral or word columns. This pattern is seen on spelling papers and in arithmetic problems. If the columns are uneven, with units spreading apart and zig-zagging down the page, faulty vision is usually to blame.

Score Sheet—JVST—Jordan Vision Screening Test

Name_____ Date_____
                                            year   month   day
Present Grade_____   Birthdate _____
                                            year   month   day
Intelligence __   __   __   Age _____
          low average high   years   months
Dominance: Eye___   ___   Hand___   ___   Foot___   ___
          left   right   left   right   left   right

Instructions for Scoring

On Checklists 1, 2, 3, and 4, mark every symptom you observe in the student's visual performance. Add up the points in parentheses for every item checked. This yields the TOTAL SCORE below.

TOTAL SCORE: ____ 0-4   No serious problem. Should have little difficulty with sustained reading or writing.

____ 5-9   Visual problems exist. Student might be able to compensate if taught how to work around problems. Referral to vision specialist may prove necessary.

____ 10-14   Referral should be made to vision specialist. Student will have difficulty with reading and writing. Must be given consideration and taught how to cope in the classroom.

Must learn to pace self to avoid frustration and visual fatigue.

____ 15 or higher — Serious visual limitations. Referral should be made to vision specialist. Student cannot cope with classroom pressures without assistance.

Referred to_____ Date_____

Results of Referral _____

Test 1—Convergence at Near Point

(1) ____Eyes widen as target approaches nose

(2) ____Target blurs, goes fuzzy, or otherwise goes in and out of focus as it approaches nose

(2) ____Student pulls head back or tries to lean away from approaching target

(2) ____Student complains of headache, eye ache, or other discomfort as target moves toward nose

(1) ____Target doubles at certain points between wrist and elbow

(1) ____Target disappears at certain points between wrist and elbow

(2) ____One eye turns inward, outward, upward, or downward away from focal point

(1) ____Eyes water during sustained visual concentration

Total _____

Test 2—Target Pursuit at Near Point

(2) ____Eyes cannot track up-and-down, side-to-side, or follow target through arc

(1) ____Eyes flicker or "dance" as target moves through arc

(1) ____Eyes squint or widen during tracking

(2) ____Student leans back or sideways during tracking

(2) ____Student rolls head to one side during tracking

(2) ____Student cannot hold head still during tracking; head follows target instead of eyes turning

(1) ____Target blurs or goes out of focus at certain points during tracking

(2) ____Student peers at an angle to see target
(1) ____Student is surprised, utters exclamation during tracking
(1) ____Eyes water during tracking

Total _____

Test 3—Saccadic Control in Oral Reading

(1) ____Oral reading is choppy, irregular
(2) ____Student skips letters, syllables, or whole words, especially in smaller print
(1) ____Student overshoots, then jerks eyes back to correct mistakes
(2) ____In making the return sweep, student's eyes land above or below the line he should be reading
(2) ____Student needs to mark place with finger, card, or pencil
(1) ____Comprehension scores are usually lower than vocabulary scores
(1) ____Student miscalls familiar words from one place on the page to another
(2) ____Sustained reading becomes jumbled and incoherent as visual control deteriorates
(2) ____Eyes begin to water as student reads
(2) ____Student squints or widens eyes while reading
(1) ____Student rubs or brushes at eyes while reading
(2) ____Eyes grow red as reading progresses
(2) ____When student sees an unknown word, eyes dart all about page
(2) ____Student shifts posture during reading (leans close to desk; holds book close to eyes; peers sideways at book)
(1) ____Student lifts eyes from page frequently to glance about

Total _____

Test 4—Convergence Control in Handwriting

(1) ____Eyes separate while writing along the line; one eye trails
(1) ____In right-handed child, pencil grip is unusual with point downward or back toward body
(1) ____Writing pressure is dark and smeared
(2) ____Eyes have difficulty staying coordinated with pencil and hand movements during writing

(1) ____Letters and/or numerals are formed unevenly, usually larger than normal

(1) ____Writing wobbles up and down, cutting through lines

(2) ____Spacing is uneven and irregular between letters and words

(2) ____Margins are wobbly and zig-zag as columns progress down the page

(2) ____Quality of writing deteriorates after first line or two

(1) ____Quality deteriorates, then improves, as student writes down a column

Total _____

Glossary

There is a pattern of word derivation in clinical terms related to learning disabilities. The prefix a– usually denotes a complete or total condition, as in *alexia,* which means complete inability to read. The prefix dys– usually denotes a partial inability, or a partial ability, to function in the area. For example, *dyslexia* means a partial reading ability, or a partial loss of reading ability. This word structure pattern will help the reader to interpret various terms which may not be in his speaking vocabulary.

ACALCULIA.   Inability to process arithmetic symbols; inability to comprehend the abstract concepts represented by concrete numerals; inability to relate concepts to number symbols.

AGNOSIA.   Inability to recall specific sound-symbol relationships; inability to remember concepts, or to recall the concepts represented by letter forms, whole words, or other language units.

AGRAPHIA.   Inability to encode in written form; inability to remember how to write alphabet symbols; inability to write legibly even when specific symbols are clearly in view.

ALEXIA.   Inability to decode printed word symbols; inability to read after considerable exposure to educational techniques for teaching reading.

ANOXIA.   Temporary loss of oxygen in important centers of the brain; usually results in brain damage which may cause learning difficulties.

APHASIA.   Inability to use language coherently or meaningfully; inability to correlate concepts with word symbols, or to recall concepts represented by word units.

AUDITORY DYSLEXIA.   Difficulty encoding (translating) speech into printed or written symbols; difficulty identifying ("hearing") discrete phonic elements of speech accurately; difficulty making sound-symbol associations.

BRADYSLEXIA.   Extremely slow rate of reading, writing, or spelling.

CYLERT.   (Pemoline) A stimulant drug used to control the symptoms of hyperkinesis. Often used in conjunction with Valium. Usually administered once daily in the morning.

DEXEDRINE. A stimulant drug used to control the symptoms of hyper-kinesis. Seldom as effective as Ritalin or Cylert.

DYSCALCULIA. Difficulty learning to process arithmetic symbols; partial ability (or inability) to comprehend the relationships between math concepts and symbols.

DYSGNOSIA. Difficulty remembering specific concept-symbol relation-ships; partial ability (or inability) to remember which concepts are represented by specific symbols.

DYSGRAPHIA. Difficulty putting thoughts into written form; partial ability (or inability) to remember how to make certain alphabet or arithmetic symbols in handwriting; involves faulty sense of direc-tionality (left to right; top to bottom).

DYSLEXIA. Difficulty processing language symbols; partial ability (or inability) to decode printed symbols into thought, or to encode thought into printed or written symbols.

ECHOLALIA. Tendency to subvocalize (mutter, whisper, move lips) while reading or writing; tendency to transpose syllables when re peating word units (alunimum for aluminum).

ENDOPHASIA. Tendency for listener to move his lips in time with speaker's voice.

HYPERACTIVITY. Habitual nervous, jittery behavior which can be con-trolled by child, but which is a distracting factor in learning situations; responds to tranquilizing drug therapy; similar to but not the same as hyperkinesis.

HYPERKINESIS. Nervous, jittery, destructive, disruptive, abrasive behav-ior which child cannot control; responds to stimulant drug therapy, but not to tranquilizing drugs (see Minimal Cerebral Dysfunction).

HYPOKINESIS. Sluggish, surly, self-centered, antisocial behavior; usu-ally accompanied by obesity; infantile emotional reactions cause chronic social conflict.

IDEATIONAL AGNOSIA. Inability to visualize or recall constructions of words; inability to remember which letters are needed for correct spellings; difficulty in recalling correct order (sequence) of letters within words; handwriting may be clearly legible, but content does not make sense.

INVERSION. Turning letters upside down within words while reading or writing (way for may   yelp for help).

LEGASTHENIA. Inability to relate ideas (concepts) to symbols (percepts); a bridge is out between ideas (experience) and the symbols representing the ideas.

MINIMAL BRAIN DYSFUNCTION. An umbrella term used for a variety of disabilities; a general term used when a child cannot read at all (alexia), or can partially read, write, or spell (dyslexia); occasionally used to designate aphasia or dysphasia.

MINIMAL CEREBRAL DYSFUNCTION. Often a synonym for hyperkinesis.

MINIMAL CUES. The small details which differentiate symbols from each other; small details in writing or printing (capitals, punctuation marks, indention, etc.).

MIRROR IMAGE. Tendency to perceive from right to left.

MIRROR READING. Tendency to read words or number groups backwards (was for saw   no for on   37 for 73).

MIRROR WRITING. Tendency to start from right side and write toward the left; often entire words are reversed as if seen in a mirror.

MOTOR AGNOSIA. Inability to write legible letter or word forms; handwriting resembles a series of scratches, although the writer may have a clear mental image of how the letter forms should appear; the handwriting often makes sense to the writer, but is illegible to others.

ORAL APHASIA. Inability to enunciate or say the words intended; sometimes referred to as *motor oligophasia*.

ORIENTATION REVERSAL. Perceiving or writing symbols backward; same as *mirror image*.

PERSEVERATION. Tendency to run on and on while speaking, writing, or spelling; inability to turn loose of one pattern in order to begin a new one (edgege for edge   banananana for banana   Kent Keng for Kent King).

PLEONASM. Tendency to add unnecessary words in oral or written language; tendency to add words to text while reading or copying.

PRIMARY READING DISABILITY. Reading failure because of organic, emotional, or perceptual disability.

PRINTER'S CUES. Nonlanguage cues used by printer to highlight or emphasize particular points on a page (color bands, underlining, italics, boldface type, indentation).

REVERSAL. Changing position of letters, syllables, or sound units within words (paly for play aet for ate); also used to refer to turning letters backward (b for d).

RITALIN. Medication given for control of hyperkinesis; a form of "speed" (amphetamine class of drugs) which is not habit forming in hyperkinetics; side effects are sometimes seen (insomnia, constipation, decreased appetite, drop in white cell count in blood test); cancels out the violent impulses of hyperkinetic behavior, allowing the child to concentrate and change his attitudes toward school.

ROTATION. Turning around certain letter forms within words (deb for bed tup for tub mnst for must).

SACCADIC. The eye movement rhythms involved in reading as the eyes work together focusing from point to point along a line of print. Faulty eye muscle balance makes smooth saccadics impossible to achieve without visual correction.

SECONDARY READING DISABILITY. Reading failure because of poor teaching, faulty attention, lack of application, faulty vision, poor health, and so on.

SEMANTIC APHASIA. Pronouncing or repeating words correctly without comprehending their meanings; often seen when children can decode fluently but have no idea of what they have just read.

SPECIFIC DYSLEXIA. Often used to designate specific reading disabilities which have been identified or analyzed.

SUBSTITUTION. Mentally or physically replacing one letter or word with another while reading or writing (bottle for battle run for ran); also refers to failure to observe minimal cues, such as minor details that distinguish similar letter forms, punctuation cues, printer's cues, and so forth.

TELESCOPING. Omitting portions of words in reading or spelling; running letters together in writing (dghse for doghouse pecl for pencil).

TRANSPOSING. Placing or perceiving letters or numerals in wrong positions while reading or writing.

VISUAL DYSLEXIA. Difficulty interpreting ("seeing") printed or written symbols accurately; tendency to perceive symbols upside down, backwards, or in scrambled sequence; inability to comprehend items presented in series.

VISUAL AGNOSIA.   Inability to perceive overall configurations; the reader sees only isolated symbols instead of clusters, syllables, whole word units, or whole number units.

VISUAL APHASIA.   Inability to recognize printed words as representing the person's listening-speaking vocabulary; inability to comprehend the fact that print is talk written down; sometimes a synonym for *legasthenia*.

Index